MEDICAL MYCOLOGY MANUAL

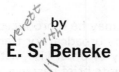

by

E. S. Beneke

Department of Botany and Plant Pathology
College of Natural Science
and
Department of Microbiology and Public Health
College of Human Medicine

Michigan State University

and

A. L. Rogers

Department of Botany and Plant Pathology
College of Natural Science

Michigan State University

Third Edition

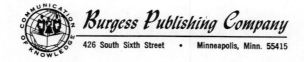

Burgess Publishing Company

426 South Sixth Street • Minneapolis, Minn. 55415

Copyright © 1970, 1966, 1957 by E. S. Beneke
Printed in the United States of America
SBN-8087-0263-7

3 4 5 6 7 8 9 0

PREFACE TO THE FIRST EDITION

This manual is primarily intended for use by laboratory technicians, microbiologists, and other students in medical mycology courses as a guide in the study and laboratory identification of pathogenic fungi in men and animals. For more detailed information on symptomology, pathology, differential diagnosis, prognosis and treatment, reference should be made to textbooks or references.

The material in this manual has been arranged so that the student trained in bacteriological procedures, with little or no training in mycology is introduced to some of the essential characteristics of fungi and some of the common contaminants before handling any of the pathogenic fungi. Subsequent to becoming acquainted with some of the common contaminants, it has been found that the student receives valuable training while trying to isolate and identify as many unknown fungi as possible on culture media from various sources such as air borne spores, dust in attics, soil or dung.

Most of the pathogenic fungi that have been reported to occur as clinical cases in North America are included in this manual. Some of the fungus diseases included in this manual are usually found to be more prevalent in other parts of the world, but may occur in North America when people travel so rapidly from one continent to another. Each disease contains information on type of material that may contain the fungus, procedures for direct microscopic examination of the material, staining technics, culture procedures, macroscopic appearance of the organism if grown in culture, microscopic appearance of the fungus, histological studies and animal inoculation procedures where applicable. A selection of some of the current references are included for additional information on technics and mycological aspects of the organism. This manual has been arranged so that the student or the medical technician can readily refer to the essential characteristics of each disease which should aid in a more rapid laboratory diagnosis of the etiological agent.

PREFACE TO THE THIRD EDITION

Since the publication of the first edition of the *Medical Mycology Laboratory Manual* thirteen years ago, many changes have occurred in the field of medical mycology. New culture media, improved immunological methods, use of fluorescent antibody techniques, and methods for physiological differentiation have aided in more accurate identification of pathogens. More specific stains have been used in recent years to distinguish fungi in fixed tissue and slide preparations. Many of these changes have been incorporated in this edition.

An increase in fungal diseases is taking place in recent years as a result of the use of broad spectrum antibiotics for treatment of bacterial diseases and from the use of chemotherapeutic agents for treatment of different types of malignancies. The need for specific identification of the etiologic agent is of greater importance in such cases.

In the third edition new color plates have been added. These include illustrations of the different types of dermatomycoses and the various dermatophytes. It is hoped that added color illustrations of a number of colonies of *Microsporum* spp., *Epidermophyton* sp., and *Trichophyton* spp. may make laboratory identification of this group easier. It is important to remember that color and morphological characteristics of colonies will vary in different isolates.

Better differentiation and determination of the pathogenic fungi in recent years have been greatly aided by the development of improved techniques. Some of these techniques increase the rapidity and accuracy of identification of these fungi.

An index has been added for the convenience of the user.

Additions to the manual include torulopsosis, streptotrichosis, and keratomycosis. These diseases have been reported more frequently in recent years. Streptotrichosis, an actinomycete is frequently identified in the medical mycology laboratory and has been included in this edition. It is primarily a disease of animals although occasionally a few spontaneous infections have been reported in humans.

November 1970

E. S. Beneke, Ph.D.
A. L. Rogers, Ph.D.

ACKNOWLEDGEMENTS

The authors are most grateful to the Upjohn Company staff, especially to Baird Thomas, Editor, and A. Garrard Macleod, M.D., Consultant, for making arrangements to publish the original color slides in *Scope Monograph on Human Mycoses* by E. S. Beneke. They also wish to express appreciation to Mr. Baird A. Thomas, and Mr. Paul Duensing, Special Projects Department, The Upjohn Company, for reprinting the original color plates, three folded inserts, and the color separation for the cover of the third edition of this manual.

Through the kindness of Miss Mary Ellen Hopper we were able to use Figures 51-70, 73-76, 78-88 and 90 to illustrate the dermatomycoses. These slides were taken by the late George Lewis, M.D. Harold Van Velsor, M.D., Wilmington, North Carolina provided the illustrations of tinea nigra. We are also indebted to A. P. Ulbrich, D.O. for making available some of the photographs of the dermatomycoses. The authors wish to express appreciation to Thomas S. Turner, Cytologist, B.P.A., of the Department of Gynecology and Obstetrics, New Jersey College of Medicine and Dentistry, Jersey City, New Jersey for the slide of hyphae and spores of *Candida* species.

The authors are also indebted to the late Dr. Emma S. Moss, Director, Department of Pathology, Charity Hospital of Louisiana, and Dr. Albert L. McQuown, Pathologist, Our Lady of the Lake Sanitarium, Baton Rouge, Louisiana for permission to use the photographs of the deep mycoses published in the *Scope Monograph on Human Mycoses,* and to Dr. Arthur E. Schultz, East Lansing, Michigan for use of the photograph of Aspergillosis infection in the eye.

The authors are indebted to Patrick Bourke, Instructor, Port Huron Junior College, Port Huron, Michigan for making the illustrations.

The inspiration and encouragement of Dr. Const. J. Alexopoulos and Dr. C. W. Emmons have been greatly appreciated during the preparation of the first edition of the manual. Much appreciation has been expressed to Claire Taschdjian for taking time to examine the original manuscript of the first edition. Some of the original slide cultures used for photomicrographs were prepared with the able assistance of Mrs. Mary E. Joy Matson. The acquaintance and association with Dr. N. F. Conant and others in the field of medical mycology has been an inspiration in the study and teaching of medical mycology.

The authors are indebted to many colleagues and students for suggestions in the development and in the revisions of the manual.

E. S. Beneke

A. L. Rogers

CONTENTS

CHARACTERISTICS OF FUNGI

Introduction

In order to become acquainted with some of the fungi among many thousands in the world, an introduction to a systematic arrangement of these organisms is a necessity. After the introduction of a few basic concepts on terminology, the major classification system, and a few organisms, the identification of fungi becomes much easier. After becoming acquainted with some of the contaminants and the pathogenic fungi, the medical bacteriologists, medical technologists, physicians, and veterinarians will have a better concept about the behavior of fungi when pathogenic in man or animals.

Fungi have somatic or vegetative structures that may be one-celled or tubular in form. These tubes or threads are known as *hyphae* or a single thread is a *hypha*. The hyphae branch and may have cross-walls or *septa*. The hyphae develop from spores which vary considerably in one organism or another. A large mat of hyphal growth is known as *mycelium*.

Two general types of reproduction occur in the fungi: asexual and sexual. Asexual reproduction is the most common in the pathogenic fungi which in most cases do not reproduce sexually. Asexual reproduction may be by (1) fragmentation of hyphae, (2) breaking up of cells in the hyphae into their component cells which are called arthrospores (oidia), (3) cells may become thick-walled and are known as chlamydospores, (4) while the most common type of asexual reproduction is by means of spores. Yeasts may multiply by budding (blastospores) or by cell division.

Classification

The same categories or groupings that apply to other plants as a means of classification and separation of the organisms also apply to fungi. The categories include: Kingdom, Division, Class, Order, Family, Genus, and Species. Although there are variations in classification systems, there are usually four classes considered (unless the Phycomycetes are split into six separate classes) in the true fungi or Eumycotina:

1. *Phycomycetes* includes a number of one-celled organisms, but most of the group are filamentous. The mycelium usually lacks cross-walls, and the organisms reproduce asexually by means of sporangia which contain motile or nonmotile spores, by sporangioles, or by conidia. Sexual reproduction results in formation of a thick-walled resting spore such as a zygospore or öospore. Only a few pathogens occur in this group.

2. *Ascomycetes* have cross-walls or septa in the mycelium. Asexual reproduction varies from budding cells, cell division, breaking up of cells in the hyphae, to a specialized branch or conidiophore bearing conidia.

3. *Basidiomycetes* have septate hyphae with uninucleate or binucleate cells. The binucleate mycelium which arises from sexual reproduction usually forms clamp connections or bulges on the side of the cells where the nuclei divide in the formation of new cells. The typical reproductive structure is the basidium, a club-shaped structure usually bearing 4 basidiospores on the surface. This group is of little importance in causing human or animal diseases. At times mushroom poisoning is of importance in medical practice.

4. *Deuteromycetes* (Fungi Imperfecti) is an artificial group of fungi which reproduce by asexual means only. Many apparently would be Ascomycetes or in some cases Basidiomycetes if the sexual stage were found to occur. Most of the pathogenic fungi in man and animals belong to this class.

RELATIONSHIP OF VARIOUS CATEGORIES OF THE FUNGI

CLASS	Sub-Class, Series, or Order	Examples of Genera or Species
Myxomycetes (Slime molds)	6 Orders	

Schizomycetes (Bacteria) — *Higher bacteria*:

Eubacterials (true bacteria) .... Corynebacterium tenuis

Actinomycetales (funguslike bacteria; may branch) } Actinomyces, Nocardia, Streptomyces

Chlamydobacteriales (algalike bacteria; may be sheathed)

Myxobacteriales (slime bacteria; slimy creeping mass)

Spirochaetales (protozoalike bacteria)

Rickettsiales (intracellular parasites)

Lower fungi

Phycomycetes (algal fungi; nonseptate hyphae; asexual spores formed in sporangia: oöspores or zygospores formed sexually)

Chytridiales .... (?) Rhinosporidium (uniflagellate zoospores)

Saprolegniales—sexual: oöspores .... (water molds) (Biflagellate zoospores)

Mucorales—sexual: zygospores .... (Nonmotile spores)

Rhizopus [Bread mold] —(sporangia at nodes of stolons opposite Rhizoids)

Mucor — (sporangia directly on mycelium; no rhizoids)

Absidia

Higher fungi

Ascomycetes (sac fungi; form ascospores, typically 8, sexually in an ascus or sac)

Sub-Class Hemiascomycetidae Endomycetales (yeasts)

Sub-class Euascomycetidae

Series Plectomycetes—3 orders .... (cleistothecia, black molds, blue molds)

Arthroderma, Nannizzia, Allescheria } Dermatophyte Perfect Stage

Series Pyrenomycetes—9 orders .... Piedraia (the perithecial fungi)

Series Discomycetes—4 orders (cup fungi, morels, and truffles)

Form-Class Deuteromycetes (imperfect fungi; asexual stages of Ascomycetes or rarely Basidiomycetes whose sexual stages are yet undiscovered)

Form-Order Melanconiales (reproduce by conidia in acervuli)

Form-Order Sphaeropsidales (reproduce by conidia in pycnidia)

Form-Order Moniliales .... (reproduce by conidia borne otherwise, or by oidia, or by budding)

Aspergillus	Histoplasma
Blastomyces	Keratinomyces
Candida	Madurella
Cephalosporium	Malassezzia
Cladosporium	Microsporum
Coccidioides	Paracoccidioides
Cryptococcus	Phialophora
Epidermophyton	Sporotrichum
Fonsecaea	Trichophyton
Geotrichum	Trichosporon

Basidiomycetes (produce sexual spores on a base, or basidium)

Sub-class Heterobasidiomycetidae—3 orders (jelly fungi, rusts, smuts)

Sub-class Homobasidiomycetidae—8 orders (mushrooms, puffballs, shelf, coral, and bird's nest fungi)

In order to develop a better background concerning fungi, it is suggested that reference be made to a textbook on mycology such as *Introductory Mycology* by Const. J. Alexopoulos. There are a number of other reference books or textbooks that may be utilized in the study of fungi.

Selected References in General Mycology

1. AINSWORTH, G. C. and G. R. Bisby. 1961. Dictionary of Fungi. 5th Edition. Commonwealth Mycological Institute, Kew, Surrey, England.
2. ALEXOPOULOS, C. J. 1962. Introductory Mycology. 2nd Edition. John Wiley & Sons, Inc., New York.
3. ALEXOPOULOS, C. J. and E. S. Beneke. 1962. Laboratory Manual for Introductory Mycology. Burgess Publishing Co., Minneapolis.
4. BARNETT, H. L. 1960. Illustrated Genera of Imperfect Fungi. 2nd Edition. Burgess Publishing Co., Minneapolis.
5. BARRON, GEORGE L. 1968. The Genera of Hyphomycetes from Soil. The Williams & Wilkins Co., Baltimore.
6. BESSEY, E. A. 1950. Morphology and Taxonomy of Fungi. The Blakiston Co., Philadelphia.
7. BURNETT, J. H. 1968. Fundamentals of Mycology. St. Martin's Press, New York.
8. CLEMENTS, F. E. and C. L. Shear. 1931. Genera of Fungi. The H. W. Wilson Co., New York.
9. GAUMANN, E. A. 1952. The Fungi. (Transl. by F. L. Wynd.) Hafner Publishing Co., New York.
10. GILMAN, J. C. 1957. A Manual of Soil Fungi. The Iowa State University Press, Ames.
11. RAPER, K. B. and C. Thom. 1949. A Manual of the Penicillia. The Williams and Wilkins Co., Baltimore.
12. RAPER, K. B. and D. F. Fennell. 1965. The Genus Aspergillus. The Williams & Wilkins Co., Baltimore.

Selected Reference Books in Medical Mycology

1. AINSWORTH, G. C. 1952. Medical Mycology. An Introduction to Its Problems. Sir Isaac Pitman & Sons, Ltd., London, England.
2. AINSWORTH, G. C. and P. K. C. Austwick. 1958. Fungal Diseases of Animals. Commonwealth Agricultural Bureaux. Farnham Royal, England.
3. AJELLO, L., L. K. Georg, W. Kaplan and L. Kaufman. 1963. Laboratory Manual for Medical Mycology. PHSP No. 994. Superintendent of Documents, U. S. Government Printing Office. Washington 25, D.C.
4. BENEKE, E. S. 1969. Scope Monograph on Human Mycoses. The Upjohn Co., Kalamazoo, Michigan.
5. CIFERRI, R. 1960. Manuale di Micologia Medica. I, II. Pavia. Casa Editrice Renzo Cortina, Italy.
6. CONANT, N. F., D. T. Smith, R. D. Baker, J. L. Callaway and D. S. Martin. 1954. Manual of Clinical Mycology. 2nd Edition. W. B. Saunders Co., Philadelphia, Pa.
7. DUBOS, R. J. and J. G. Hirsch. 1965. Bacterial and Mycotic Infections of Man. Lippincott Co. Philadelphia.
8. DVOŘAK, J. and M. Otčenašek. 1969. Mycological Diagnosis of Animal Dermatophytoses. Dr. W. Junk N. V., Publishers. The Hague.
9. EMMONS, C. W., C. H. Binford and J. P. Utz. 1963. Medical Mycology. Lea and Febiger. Philadelphia, Pa.
10. FEGELER, F. 1967. Medizinische Mykologie in Praxis und Klinik. Springer-Verlag, Berlin, Heidelberg, New York.

11. HALEY, L. D. 1964. Diagnostic Medical Mycology. Appleton-Century-Crofts. New York, N. Y.

12. HAZEN, E. S., M. A. Gordon and F. C. Reed. 1970. Laboratory Identification of Pathogenic Fungi Simplified. 3rd Edition. Charles C. Thomas. Springfield, Ill.

13. HILDICK-SMITH, G., H. Blank and I. Sarkany. 1964. Fungus Diseases and Their Treatment. Little, Brown and Co. Boston, Mass.

14. KRAL, F. 1964. Veterinary Dermatology. Lippincott Co. Philadelphia.

15. LANGERON, M. and R. Vanbreuseghem. 1952. Précis de mycologie. Masson et Cie edit., Paris.

16. LACAZ, C. S. 1967. Compêndio de Micologia Médica. Sarvier, Editora de Livros Médicos, Ltda, São Paulo.

17. LEWIS, G. M., M. E. Hopper, J. W. Wilson and O. A. Plunkett. 1958. An Introduction to Medical Mycology. 4th Edition. The Year Book Publishers, Inc. Chicago, Ill.

18. MOSS, E. S. and A. L. McQuown. 1969. Atlas of Medical Mycology. 3rd Edition. Williams and Wilkins Co., Baltimore, Maryland.

19. NEGRONI, P. (Translated by S. McMillen.) 1965. Histoplasmosis, Diagnosis and Treatment. Revised Edition. Charles C. Thomas, Springfield, Ill.

20. REBELL, G., D. Taplin and H. Blank. 1964. Dermatophytes, Their Recognition and Identification. Dermatology Foundation of Miami, 1020 N. W. 16th St., Miami, Fla.

21. RIPPON, John. 1969. Chapter 32. Medical Mycology: The pathogenic fungi and the pathogenic actinomycetes. In W. Burrows: Textbook of Microbiology, the Pathogenic Microorganisms. 19th Edition. W. B. Saunders Co. Philadelphia.

22. SABOURAUD, R. 1910. Les Teignes. Masson and Cie. Paris, France.

23. SEGRETAIN, G., E. Drouhet and F. Mariat. 1964. Le Diagnostic de Laboratoire en Mycologie Médicale. 2e édit. La Tourelle.

24. SIMMONS, R. D. G., Ph. (Editor). 1954. Medical Mycology. Cleaver-Hume Press Ltd., London, England.

25. SMITH, D. T., N. F. Conant and H. P. Willett. 1968. Zinsser Microbiology, section on Medical Mycology by N. F. Conant, pp 1085-1186. 14th Edition. Appleton-Century-Crofts, New York.

26. STERNBERG, T. H. and V. D. Newcomer. 1955. Therapy of Fungus Diseases. Little, Brown and Co., Boston, Mass.

27. SWEANY, H. C. (Editor). 1960. Histoplasmosis. Charles C. Thomas, Springfield, Ill.

28. VANBREUSEGHEM, R. and J. Wilkinson. 1958. Mycoses of Man and Animals. Sir Isaac Pitman and Sons, Ltd., London.

29. VANBREUSEGHEM, R. 1966. Guide Pratique de Mycologie Médicale et Vétérinaire. Masson et Cie, Paris.

30. WILSON, J. W. 1957. Clinical and Immunological Aspects of Fungous Disease. Charles C. Thomas, Springfield, Ill.

31. WILSON, J. W. and O. A. Plunkett. 1965. The Fungous Diseases of Man. University of California Press, Berkeley and Los Angeles, Calif.

32. WINNER, H. I. and R. Hurley. 1964. *Candida Albicans.* Little, Brown and Co. Boston, Mass.

33. ZAPATER, R. C. 1956. El Diagnóstico Micológico de Laboratorio. El Ateneo, Buenos Aires.

Scientific Periodicals, Abstracts, and Memoranda

1. Mycologia. Lancaster Press, Lancaster, Pa.

2. Mycopathologia et Mycologia Applicata. Dr. W. Junk, 13 van Stolkweg. The Hague, Netherlands.

3. Mykosen, Organ für Experimentelle und Klinische Mykologie. Berliner Medizinische Verlagsantalt. Berlin-Lichterfelde-West. Baseler Strasse 67.

4. Medical Mycology Committee (J. T. Ingram, Chairman). 1967. Nomenclature of fungi pathogenic to man and animals. Memorandum No 23. Third Edition. Medical Research Council. Her Majesty's Stationery Office. London.

5. Review of Medical and Veterinary Mycology. 1943 to date. Commonwealth Mycological Institute, Kew, Surrey, England. (Abstracts in medical mycology.)
6. Sabouraudia. Journal of the International Society for Human and Animal Mycology. E. and S. Livingstone, Ltd., Edinburgh and London.

In addition to these references, numerous articles may be found in the various medical journals and in certain biological science journals.

A SUGGESTED LABORATORY SCHEDULE

The following schedule is based on two-hour laboratory periods. This may be of special aid to the instructor who is beginning to teach medical mycology for the first time. Additional demonstrations, materials, and audiovisual aids are useful when available (see sources of materials in the back of the manual). Whenever possible the following fungi should be grown on slide cultures for mounts and in bottle or plate cultures for study by the students (exceptions: *Coccidioides immitis*, *Histoplasma capsulatum*, and possibly a few other systemic fungi for slide cultures).

LABORATORY PERIOD	ORGANISMS FOR STUDY
1	Introduction, equipment needed. Demonstration of slide culture method. Start slide culture of *Aspergillus* sp.; *Penicillium* sp.; *Gliocladium* sp.; and *Scopulariopsis* sp. Direct mounts and tape mounts from cultures.
2	Start slide culture of *Trichoderma* sp.; and *Geotrichum* sp. Make tape mounts of the above fungi; identify the structures. Bring organic soil samples for the next period.
3	Complete slide culture demonstration. Start slide cultures of *Cladosporium* sp.; *Fusarium* sp.; *Cephalosporium* sp.; *Nigrospora* sp. Start hair-baiting technique with soil samples for isolation of keratinophilic fungi.
4	Start slide cultures of *Alternaria* sp.; *Helminthosporium* sp. Review all contaminants studied on self-study projector screen, slide cultures, and tube cultures. Expose plates to dust samples or airborne fungus spores. Culture media, isolation techniques.
5	Start slide culture of *Syncephalastrum* sp. Optional slide cultures: *Mucor* sp.; *Aureobasidium pullulans (Pullularia pullulans)*. Unknowns.
6	Direct mounts: *Streptomyces* sp.; *Rhodotorula* sp. Start *Trichophyton* sp. on Trichophyton agars. Inoculate mice with soil samples that may contain systemic fungi. Complete slide cultures of contaminants. Check identification of contaminants in exposed plates.
7	Complete identification of genera in exposed plates; review all contaminants on self-study screen, slides, and tube cultures.
8	Demonstrations and cultures of *Piedraia hortai* and *Trichosporon beigelii*. Stain *Malassezia furfur* in skin scrapings by the periodic acid-Schiff stain method after fixing to slide.
9	Methods for culture of dermatophytes; check soil cultures for presence of keratinophilic fungi and isolate positive hairs on Sabouraud agar with antibiotics. Use of Wood's light for positive *Microsporum* hair infections. Start slide cultures of *Microsporum audouinii*, *M. gypseum*, *M. cookei*, and *M. nanum*. Check culture display of dermatophytes.
10	Start other dermatophyte slide cultures. Review the dermatophyte cultures and microscopic characteristics on the self-study projector screen. Unknowns.
11	Mount slide cultures of *Microsporum* sp. when ready. Study *Microsporum canis*; *Epidermophyton floccosum* cultures. Culture fungus from skin, nail, or hair of a patient. Check for the presence of fungi in skin or nail by the KOH method. Check the growth patterns on the Trichophyton agars. Make a direct mount of *M. ferrugineum*.

ORGANISMS FOR STUDY

12	Mount slide cultures of *Trichophyton mentagrophytes; T. rubrum; T. ajelloi;* and *T. tonsurans* or *T. gallinae, T. megninii* and others if set up. Direct mounts may be made of *T. schoenleinii, T. violaceum,* and *T. verrucosum.* Unknowns.
13	Film strips on dermatophytes. Movie on Griseofulvin. Review of dermatophyte cultures, slide cultures, and self-study projector screen.
14	Injection of animals with *Sporothrix schenckii; Histoplasma capsulatum; Blastomyces dermatitidis; Paracoccidioides brasiliensis;* and *Cryptococcus neoformans.* Completion of slide set.
15	Review period.
16	Spot test.
17	Start slide cultures of *Fonsecaea pedrosoi* (Syn: *Hormodendrum pedrosoi); Fonsecaea compacta* (Syn: *Hormodendrum compactum); Phialophora verrucosa.* Check tissue or pus from case of chromoblastomycosis. Start slide cultures of *Allescheria boydii* and *Phialophora jeanselmei.* Study slides of cases of maduromycosis. Start *Aspergillus fumigatus* slide culture, and study slides of cases. Inject mice or rabbits with suspension of *Candida albicans.*
18	Study *Nocardia asteroides, N. brasiliensis, Streptomyces madurae, S. pelletieri.* Check acid-fast stain, proteolytic activity, and amylolytic activity. Study *Actinomyces israelii,* conditions of growth, microscopic morphology.
19	*Candida albicans; C. tropicalis; C. pseudotropicalis; C. krusei; C. parapsilosis;* autopsy of animals with yeast infections, stain smears of infected area of animal; check chlamydospore agars, fermentations. Serum culture technique for germ tubes. Inject animals with *Coccidioides immitis.*
20	*Cryptococcus neoformans;* india ink mount. Check infected mice for presence of organism. Autopsy of mice injected with soil suspensions. Color movie on moniliasis. *Geotrichum candidum* culture, slide culture, and stained smear of sputum containing organism.
21	Demonstration slides of various deep and subcutaneous mycoses on the microscopes. Kodachromes of symptoms, tissue and culture phases of the same diseases on the self-study projector screen.
22	*Sporothrix schenckii,* slide culture mount. Stain smears from infected areas of laboratory animals. Check yeast phase. The fluorescent antibody technique.
23	*Coccidioides immitis; Rhinosporidium seeberi;* observe demonstrations of both. Make direct mount of the killed culture of *C. immitis.* Autopsy of animal; mount infected material to find stages of spherule development. Film strips on coccidioidomycosis. Color movie on "Coccidioidomycosis."
24	*Blastomyces dermatitidis; Paracoccidioides brasiliensis;* make a mount of the mycelial and yeast phase in culture. Autopsy of animal; mount infected material and examine for thick-walled budding cells. Movie.
25	*Histoplasma capsulatum.* Make a mount of the mycelial and yeast phase in culture. Make a blood smear from an infected laboratory animal and stain. Movie on histoplasmosis. Completion of slide set.
26	Reports by students on selected topics from current literature.

27   Review, using slides, cultures, and self-study projector screen.

28   Spot test.

NOTE: The systemic fungi are studied after the yeastlike fungi and actinomycetes in the sug-
         gested schedule to allow sufficient time for the tissue phase of the disease to develop in
         the experimental animals.

COMMON CONTAMINANT FUNGI
LABORATORY PROCEDURES

Introduction

In order to become acquainted with the characteristics of growth, colonies, and appearance of the somatic (or vegetative) and reproductive structures in fungi, a study of the common contaminants, utilizing some of the more readily identifiable fungi at first, is one good way to become acquainted with the handling of these organisms by the laboratory technician. The atmosphere usually contains many of the fungi that cause contamination in cultures. Some of these may occasionally cause allergies. In a few cases some of the contaminants may be confused with the pathogenic fungi. Both contaminants and pathogenic fungi may be isolated from skin lesions, sputum, or other sources of materials from a patient.

Under rare conditions, saprophytic fungi may become pathogenic and invade the tissues. These conditions may occur in patients under prolonged therapy with antibiotics or hormones, or in patients with lowered resistance suffering from cancer, diabetes, or other diseases. An "opportunistic" saprophyte should be (1) repeatedly isolated from clinical material in such cases, (2) demonstrated in the clinical material, and (3) sent to a specialist to check species identification.

The first few lectures or laboratory periods may be devoted to an introduction to the major classification systems and terminology of the fungi, utilizing specific examples to illustrate the different classes in case there is a lack of previous background in mycology.

Selected References for Study of Contaminant Fungi

1. ALEXOPOULOS, C. J. 1962. Introductory Mycology. 2nd Edition. John Wiley and Sons, Inc., New York.
2. BARNETT, H. L. 1960. Illustrated Genera of Imperfect Fungi. Burgess Publishing Co., Minneapolis, Minnesota.
3. BARRON, G. L. 1968. The Genera of Hyphomycetes from Soil. The Williams & Wilkins Co., Baltimore.
4. GILMAN, J. C. 1957. A Manual of Soil Fungi. Iowa State College Press, Ames, Iowa. Second Edition.

Laboratory Procedure for Study of Contaminant Fungi

In the laboratory study of the common contaminants the following suggestions may be of aid:

1. **Sterile Technique:** Should be used at all times.

2. **Petri Dish Cultures:** Place a small amount of hyphae or spores or both on the center of the agar medium in a petri dish using a stiff 22-gauge nichrome wire in an inoculating needle holder and observe the rate of growth, color changes, and sporulation. Sabouraud glucose agar and many other types of media will support growth of the contaminants. Observe the development of the colony over a period of several weeks, noting rate of growth, texture, pigmentation on the surface and reverse side, as well as folds or ridges on the surface. These morphological changes are important for aid in recognition of certain genera and species of contaminants and pathogens.

3. **Fungus on Test Tube Surface:** The arrangement of the asexual reproductive structures of fungal cultures that have developed against the glass surface of test tubes may be observed directly under the 10X objective of the microscope. It is necessary to know the arrangement of the conidia on the conidiophores. Usually this can be ascertained by the same method, while a slide mount disturbs the arrangements of these structures.

4. **Direct Mounts:** Using sterile technique, remove a small portion of the colony from near the center. Place material in a drop of lactophenol with or without cotton blue mounting medium. The cotton blue dye is desirable for light-colored or colorless fungi. If material is dense, tease apart with two sterile needles and add a cover slip. Examine under low magnification of the microscope, then higher magnification for smaller organisms.

5. **Cellophane Tape-cover Glass Mounts:** This method (see Endo, 1966) will keep more of the reproductive structures of the fungus intact than the direct mount method.

   a. Place a 12-mm piece of Scotch double-sided tape on the surface of the fungus colony by means of a forceps. Apply pressure gently and remove.

   b. Press the sticky side without the fungus on a cover glass. Press gently to remove bubbles.

   c. Place the cover glass over a drop of lactophenol cotton blue or other suitable mounting medium. Alcohol or surfactants added to the mounting medium help reduce bubbles.

   Note: If human or animal pathogens are not involved, the tape may be placed on the cover glass at the beginning of the procedure.

6. **Slide Culture Method:** Growing the fungus on a slide culture will result in beautiful preparations with the sporulation characteristics of the organism remaining undisturbed. For a quick observation of spore and hyphal characteristics, direct mounts of the fungus from a colony should be made in place of the slide culture technique.

   The growth of fungi in a van Tieghem cell or by various slide culture methods should be used for a more detailed study of the fungi. A good method for obtaining permanently stained slides has been published by Riddell (1950). This procedure works for most of the filamentous fungi. Briefly the method is as follows:

   a. Pour about 15 ml of melted 2% agar medium into a sterile petri dish.

   b. After solidification, mark the medium rapidly into 1-cm squares using a flamed dissecting needle or knife and a flamed glass rod.

   c. Place a bent glass rod after flaming into a sterile petri dish containing about 7-8 ml of sterile water (10% sterilized glycerin may be added). Using sterile technique, place a slide, after passing through a flame several times, on top of the bent glass rod.

   d. Lift out an agar square and place it on the flamed slide.

   e. Inoculate the four sides of the agar block with spores or mycelial fragments of the fungus to be grown.

   f. Place a flamed cover slide centrally upon the agar block (see Fig. 1).

   g. Check the culture periodically for growth and sporulation. After sporulation has occurred, two permanently stained slides may be obtained from the slide culture by proceeding as follows:

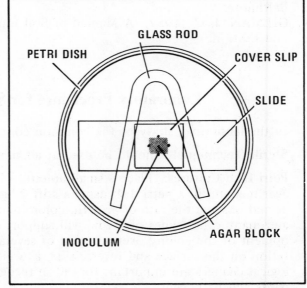

Fig. 1. Slide Culture Technique

h. Remove the cover slip from the agar block (apply a drop of 95% alcohol to the center of the cover slip in order to wet the fungus for better penetration of the mounting medium in case of *Penicillium* or *Aspergillus*).

i. Place a drop of lactophenol cotton blue on a clean slide and lower the cover slip (h) gently.

j. Similarly, using the slide with the fungus growing on it, proceed as in steps h and i, with a clean cover slip.

k. If the correct amount of mounting medium has been used, the slides may be sealed immediately with fingernail polish. The corners of the cover slip may be sealed first to hold it in position on the slide, and more lacquer may be applied after the corners are secured. In case there is excess mounting medium around the edges, it is necessary to let the slides dry overnight and then absorb the excess medium with blotting paper before sealing. These slides should keep indefinitely if well sealed. Substitutes for nail polish may be used for sealing the slides. When a slide does dry out, the nail polish may be removed from one side of the cover slip, a drop of mounting medium added, and, after filling up the dry area under the cover slip, resealed.

7. **Microscopic Examination:** Examine the slide mounts under the microscope and note the characteristic spore structures, sporangiophore or conidiophore structure if present, and mycelial characteristics for the particular fungus being studied.

Laboratory Exercise for Study of Air and Soil Borne Fungi

1. **Air-borne Fungi:** Each member of the class should select one of the following locations to expose a petri dish containing Sabouraud glucose agar (or another medium) for different periods of time:

   a. Atmosphere in building;

   b. Atmosphere outside building;

   c. Atmosphere in basement;

   d. Atmosphere in barn or chicken house;

   e. Atmosphere where crowd fills room.

2. **Soil-borne Organisms:** After using a dilution plate technique or sprinkling particles on 4 or 5 spots on the agar medium, compare types of fungi that grow from soil samples with those in the plates that contain air-borne fungi. Use the following sources for samples:

   a. High organic content in soil;

   b. Low organic content in soil;

   c. House dust;

   d. Manure from chicken house, cow or horse stable.

3. **Results:** With the aid of reference books and comparison with knowns that have been studied in class, identify the genus of as many as possible. Keep a record of the number of genera and the number of colonies that occur. After tabulating the class results of the air-borne fungi, compare with the following list of fungi that are more frequently reported in the atmosphere at various times in the year:

Alternaria sp.	*Streptomyces* sp.
Cladosporium sp. *(Hormodendrum)*	*Rhizopus* sp.
Penicillium sp.	*Phoma* sp.

Aspergillus sp.   *Trichoderma* sp.
Monilia sp.   *Chaetomium* sp.
Botrytis sp.   Unknowns
Mucor sp.   Miscellaneous

Alternaria and *Hormodendrum* have been reported as the fungi most frequently isolated from the atmosphere throughout the year. For further details on occurrence of atmospheric spores see *Allergy in Practice,* by S. M. Feinberg, or other references.

Representative Common Saprophytic Fungi

Some of the more common contaminant fungi are described on the following pages. These saprophytic fungi, often found in clinical materials, as laboratory contaminants, may in some cases become pathogenic under special conditions, and some genera resemble the pathogenic fungi. Since there are such a large number of genera and species that may be in the Fungi Imperfecti and other classes of fungi, identification to genus is sufficient for the beginner, as more training and experience is required to determine species in most cases. Recognition of some of the common genera of the contaminant fungi is sufficient as an introduction to aid in distinguishing these from pathogenic fungi.

Penicillium sp.

Colonies: Fast-growing, shades of green, blue-green or other colors, white at first, then colored after conidia mature. Surface velvety to powdery due to abundance of conidia.

Microscopic: Brushlike conidiophores or "penicillus" developed from septate hyphae. Chains of conidia, one-celled, globose to elliptical, smooth or rough, cut off from flask-shaped sterigmata (Fig. 2, 3). Various species separated on the basis of variations in branching of conidiophores, conidia, and colonial characteristics. Occasionally pathogenic.

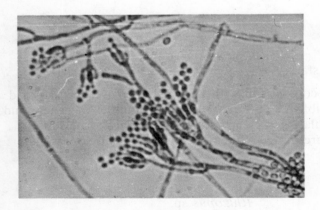

Figure 2

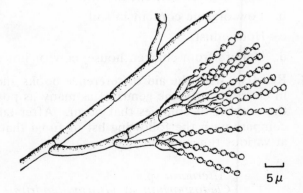

5 μ

Figure 3

Aspergillus sp.

Colonies: Slow to rapid in growth, white at first, then shades of blue-green, yellow-green, black, tan or white. Surface velvety to cottony.

Microscopic: Mycelium septate, conidiophores long with vesiclelike tip, surface containing many flask-shaped sterigmata and chains of conidia which are one-celled, spherical to elliptical, smooth or rough-walled (Fig. 4, 5). Some species develop cleistothecia (perithecia) with asci and ascospores. *A. fumigatus* pathogenic.

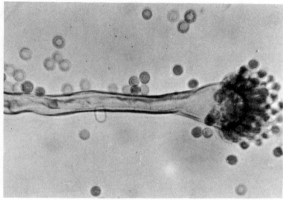

Figure 4

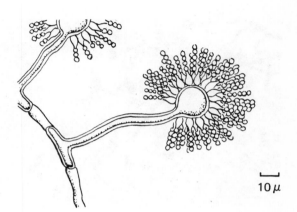

10 μ

Figure 5

Scopulariopsis sp.

Colonies: Moderately slow-growing, white at first, thin, becoming brown and powdery from heavy sporulation.

Microscopic: Mycelium septate, with single, unbranched conidiophores or branched "penicillus"-like conidiophores. Sterigmata produce chains of lemon-shaped conidia with a pointed tip and truncate base (Fig. 6, 7). Conidia usually echinulate. Occasionally in nail infections and deep-seated granulomatous lesions.

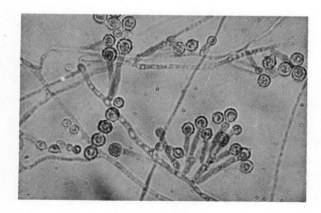

Figure 6

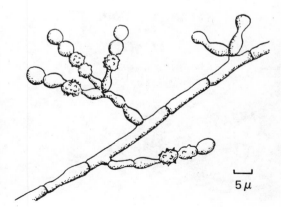

5 μ

Figure 7

Trichoderma sp.

Colonies: Fast-growing, woolly or cottony, thin, white at first, becoming green, yellow-green, or remaining white due to dense mats of conidia on surface.

Microscopic: Septate hyphae, with short, branched conidiophores, with ultimate branches flask-shaped, opposite or in whorls. Single-celled conidia formed in rounded clusters at tips of conidiophores, colorless to green (Fig. 8, 9).

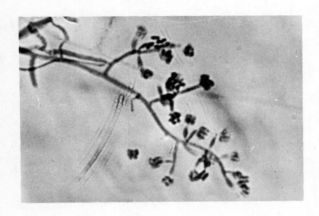

Figure 8

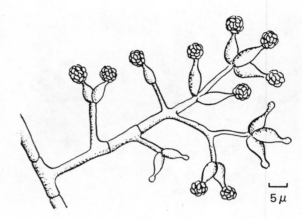

Figure 9

Paecilomyces (Spicaria) sp.

Colonies: Rather rapid growth, thin, spreading, powdery to velvety, becoming yellowish-brown, gray-green, violet or white, depending upon species.

Microscopic: Mycelium septate, with single sterigmata arising along hyphae with characteristic long tapering, conidia-bearing tubes. Also "penicillus" or *Penicillium*-like conidiophores with sterigmata having elongated tips. Conidia in chains, elliptical (Fig. 10, 11).

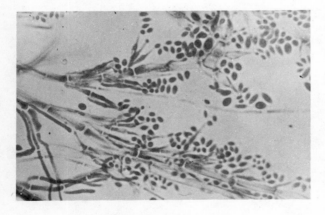

Figure 10

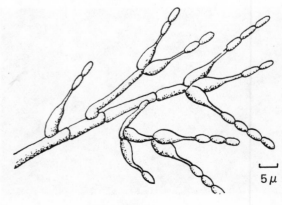

Figure 11

Gliocladium sp.

Colonies: Fast-growing, at first white, spreading over surface of plate and becoming green, rose, cream, or white.

Microscopic: Septate hyphae with conidiophores like *Penicillium,* branched with flask-shaped sterigmata at tips. Conidia one-celled, spherical, hyaline or brightly colored in mass, forming clusters or balls held together by a mucilaginous material (Fig. 12, 13). No conidial chains formed, an important distinction from *Penicillium.*

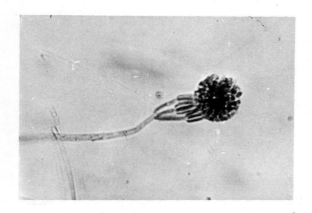

Figure 12

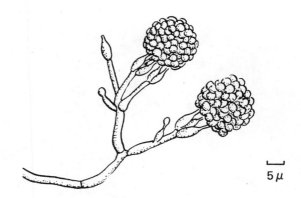

Figure 13

Cephalosporium sp.

Colonies: Fast-growing, at first compact and moist, becoming overgrown with loose, cottony aerial hyphae, white, gray, or rose in color.

Microscopic: Septate hyphae, conidiophores erect, unbranched with a cluster of conidia at the tip. Conidia elliptical, one-celled, occasionally several-celled, held together by a mucoid substance (Fig. 14, 15).

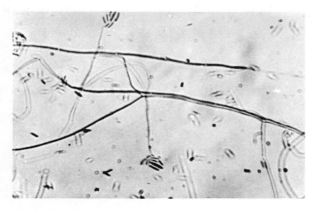

Figure 14

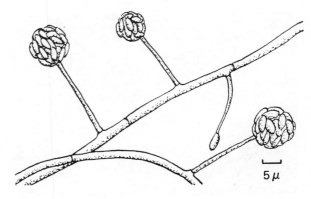

Figure 15

Fusarium sp.

    Colonies: A fast-growing fungus, at first white, cottony or woolly, frequently becoming pink, purple, or yellow in the hyphae or in the substrate.

    Microscopic: Mycelium septate, conidiophores borne singly or in packed groups (sporodochia). Conidiophores short, branched irregularly, or in whorls. Conidia of two types: macroconidia sickle-shaped, curved at the pointed ends, many-celled; microconidia one-celled, oval or elongated, some conidia two- or three-celled, elongated and curved (Fig. 16, 17). Colonies when rose in color may be confused with *Trichophyton megninii.*

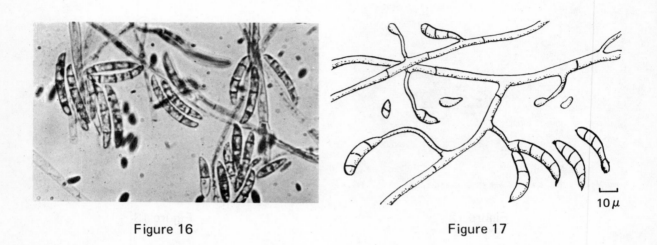

Figure 16   Figure 17

Geotrichum (Oospora) sp.

    Colonies: Fast-growing, producing cottony, aerial mycelium, white or becoming cream, tan, or greenish in color. Some species more smooth and granular on the surface on certain media.

    Microscopic: Septate hyphae, breaking up to form one-celled, thin-walled rectangular cells (arthrospores) (Fig. 18, 19). Nonpathogenic strains are commonly found in cottage cheese, rot in tomatoes, and in the soil.

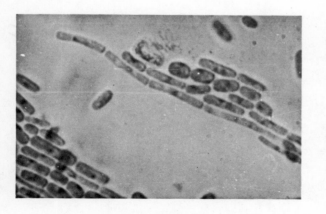
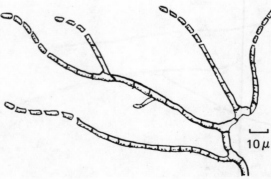

Figure 18   Figure 19

Alternaria sp.

   Colonies: Fast-growing, dense, grayish at first, becoming greenish-gray, brown, or black with gray edges. Surface overgrown with loose gray to white aerial hyphae. Reverse side of colony black.

   Microscopic: Mycelium dark, septate. Conidia produced at end of conidiophores (hyphal branches) in chains, dark brown, with transverse and longitudinal septa (muriform), variable in shape (Fig. 20, 21), with youngest conidia produced at tip of chain. *(Stemphyllium,* if conidia not in chains.)

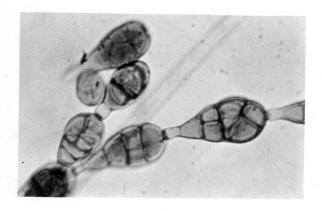

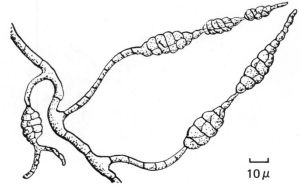

Figure 20   Figure 21

Cladosporium sp. *(Hormodendrum sp.)*

   Colonies: Moderately slow-growing, dark gray-green, reverse side brownish-gray or black. Surface powdery to velvety, becoming heaped and folded in some species.

   Microscopic: Hyphae septate, brown to olive in color; conidiophores dark, varied in length, forming branches with repeated forking, terminating in chains of conidia. Conidia one-celled (occasionally two-celled), ovate to cylindrical with pointed ends, in some cases lemon-shaped (Fig. 22, 23).

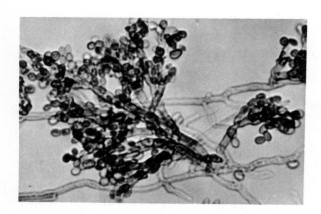

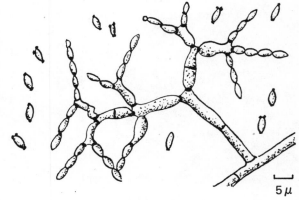

Figure 22   Figure 23

Helminthosporium sp.

Colonies: Fast-growing, grayish-brown becoming darker or black in center, velvety to woolly surface.

Microscopic: Hyphae septate, dark, with long or short, simple or branched, septate conidiophores that are twisted or bent at the tip. Conidia terminal or lateral, cylindrical to elliptical, dark, with usually more than three cells, loosely attached to the twisted or bent tip of conidiophore (Fig. 24, 25).

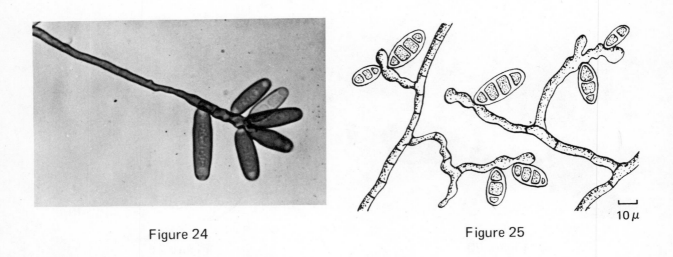

Figure 24   Figure 25

Nigrospora sp.

Colonies: Fast-growing, forming a compact cottony or woolly, white aerial mycelium becoming gray after sporulation. The reverse sides of the colonies are black.

Microscopic: Hyphae septate, with short, simple or branched, inflated conidiophores bearing jet-black, large, subspherical conidia. The vesicle or inflated tip of the conidiophore is hyaline (Fig. 26, 27).

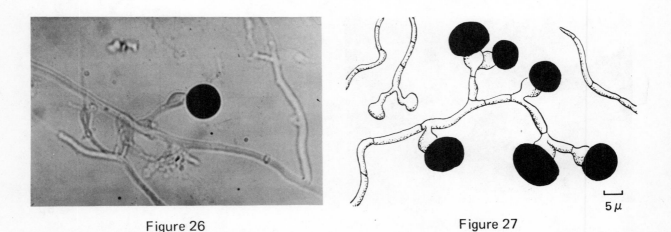

Figure 26   Figure 27

Mucor sp.

Colonies: Very fast-growing fungus quickly filling a petri plate with cottony aerial mycelium, at first white, later becoming dark gray, brown, or yellow.

Microscopic: Mycelium aseptate, forming many upright, single or branched sporangiophores. The tip of the sporangiophore bears a globose sporangium with the wall readily breaking off, leaving a collarlike base around the central columella. Spherical to elliptical spores are formed between the sporangial wall and the columella (Fig. 28, 29). No rhizoids at the base of the sporangiophores.

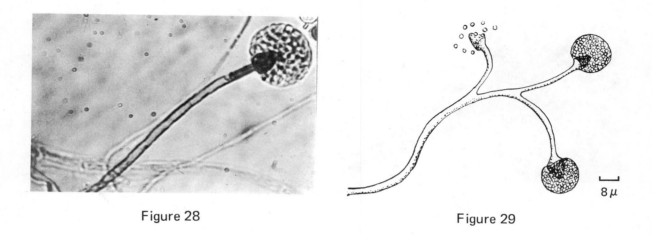

Figure 28   Figure 29

Rhizopus sp.

Colonies: Very fast-growing fungus quickly filling the culture plate with a dense cottony aerial mycelium, at first white, later becoming gray.

Microscopic: Mycelium aseptate, with many stolons (hyphal branches) connecting groups of unbranched sporangiophores. At the point of connection, a cluster of rhizoids (rootlike hyphae) are attached to the substrate. The sporangiophores terminate with a black, spherical sporangium containing a columella. Spores oval, colorless or brown (Fig. 30, 31). Zygospores formed with compatible strain.

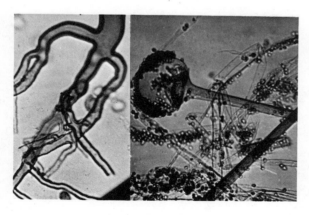

Figure 30

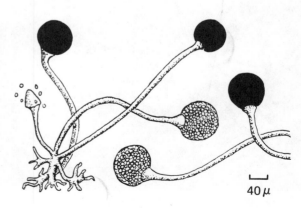

Figure 31

Syncephalastrum sp.

Colonies: Very fast-growing fungus, quickly covering the surface of the agar medium with dense, cottony, aerial mycelium which is at first white, then dark gray.

Microscopic: Mycelium aseptate, forming short sporangiophores sympodially, and terminated by an enlarged globose tip with many tubular sporangia, containing chains of spores, radiating from the globose tip. Two to many single-celled spores in each sporangium (Fig. 32, 33).

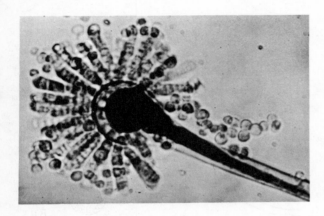

Figure 32

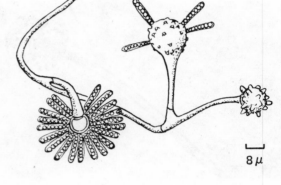

Figure 33

Aureobasidium pullulans (Pullularia pullulans)

Colonies: Young colonies at first white or pinkish and yeastlike, later becoming wrinkled, black, leathery and shiny when masses of conidia are formed.

Microscopic: Young mycelium thin-walled, producing many elliptical conidia by budding. Older hyphae are dark, thick-walled, with a short tube developed after germination to bud off elliptical conidia (Fig. 34, 35). The conidial mass makes up the shiny surface of the colony.

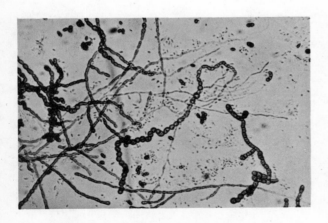

Figure 34

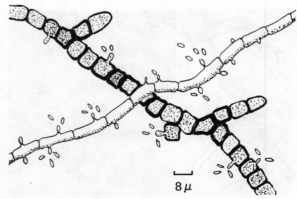

Figure 35

Rhodotorula sp.

Colonies: Yeastlike colonies develop rapidly at 37°C. The colonies are pasty, or mucoid, orange to shades of red.

Microscopic: Rather small, oval, budding yeast cells make up the colony (Fig. 36, 37). Microscopically these are similar in appearance to *Saccharomyces,* although the colony of *Saccharomyces* is cream in color.

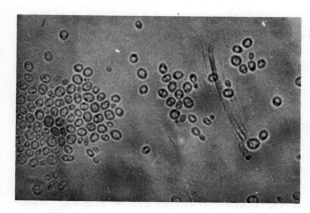

Figure 36

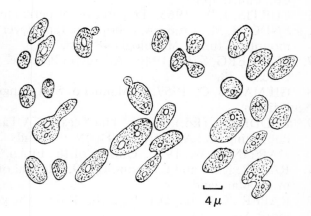

Figure 37

Streptomyces sp.

Colonies: Slow-growing, small (less than 12 mm in 14 days), dry, leathery, wrinkled, with a chalky surface, white in some species, colored in others, adherent to agar surface. Frequently with a musty odor and discoloration in the medium.

Microscopic: Thin mounts, or slide cultures, show slender (1 μ), branched hyphae with straight or coiled conidiophores breaking up into chains of conidia (Fig. 38, 39). Aerial conidia and less extensive fragmentation of hyphae help distinguish this fungus from *Nocardia.*

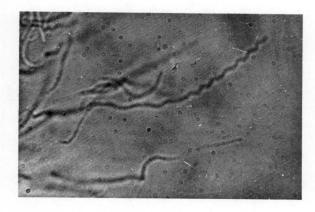

Figure 38

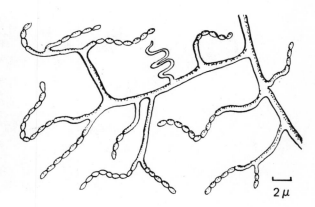

Figure 39

Additional References

1. BAKER, R. D. and E. W. Chick (Special Editors). 1962. International symposium on opportunistic fungus infections. Lab. Invest., Vol. 11, No. 11, Part 2. Williams and Wilkins Co., Baltimore, Md.

2. BESSEY, E. A. 1950. Morphology and Taxonomy of Fungi. The Blakiston Company, Philadelphia, Pa.

3. BURNETT, J. H. 1968. Fundamentals of Mycology. St. Martin's Press, New York.

4. CRIEP, L. 1967. Dermatologic Allergy: Immunology, Diagnosis, Management. W. B. Saunders Co., Philadelphia.

5. CURTIS, J. W. 1965. Preparation of permanent stained slide cultures. Archs. Derm. 91:280.

6. ENDO, R. M. 1966. A. cellophane tape-cover glass technique for preparing microscopic slide mounts of fungi. Mycologia 48:655.

7. FEINBERG, S. M. 1946. Allergy in Practice. Pp. 216-284. The Year Book Publishers, Inc. Chicago, Ill.

8. GILMAN, J. C. 1957. A Manual of Soil Fungi. Iowa State College Press, Ames, Iowa. 2nd Edition.

9. LODDER, J. (Ed.). 1970. The Yeasts — A Taxonomic Study, 2 vol. 2nd Ed. North Holland Publishing Co., Amsterdam, The Netherlands.

10. MARTIN, G. W. 1950. Outline of the Fungi. Wm. C. Brown Co., Dubuque, Iowa.

11. RAPER, K. B. and C. Thom. 1949. Manual of the Penicillia. Williams and Wilkins Co., Baltimore, Maryland.

12. RAPER, K. B. and D. F. Fennell. 1965. The genus Aspergillus. Williams and Wilkins Co., Baltimore, Maryland.

13. RIDDELL, R. W. 1950. Permanent stained mycological preparations obtained by slide culture. Mycologia 42:265.

LABORATORY PROCEDURES

Introduction

In the diagnosis of fungus infections, the most rapid method is direct examination of material on a slide to determine whether a fungus is present. If the results are negative, this does not rule out the possibility that the fungus may be missed in the sampling method. Additional procedures that may be useful in the establishment of the diagnosis are the use of: culture, Wood's light, animal inoculation, stained smears, histological sections, roentgenologic examination, immunological tests, and the fluorescent antibody technique.

Equipment

Sterilized equipment should be used at all times to avoid contamination by nonpathogenic fungi and by bacteria. The following equipment may be useful in the collection of specimens from patients.

Bard-Parker scalpel
Epilating forceps
Nail clippers
Scissors
Dental curette
Clean slides - for smears
70% alcohol
Paper packet

Syringe, 5 ml with
    18-22 gauge needles
Sterile cotton swabs
Inoculating needles
Sterile test tubes, petri
    dishes, collection bottles
Special Media
Swabs

Preparation of Specimens

The selection of proper material is important since it is difficult to know prior to microscopic examination of materials whether the fungus is in the sample selected. Selection of sufficient material for both direct examination and culture is necessary. The types of specimens collected may include: skin, nails, hair, scrapings from ulcers, pus, spinal or other body fluids, urine, sputum, blood, bone marrow, stools, bronchial washings, and biopsies (see Table I).

1. **Superficial Mycoses:** The fungi causing superficial mycoses are:

   Malassezia furfur (tinea versicolor), *Trichosporon beigelii* (white piedra), *Piedraia hortai* (black piedra), and *Cladosporium werneckii* (tinea nigra).

   For skin scrapings of tinea versicolor, the affected area should be washed with 70% alcohol to remove dirt or medication and scraped with a sterile scalpel. Place the scales in a small sterile container or a petri dish for laboratory examination.

   The same procedures are applicable for the affected areas of tinea nigra.

   In piedra cases, the hair of the scalp or beard should be cut or clipped from the areas of infection, and placed in a sterile container for laboratory examination.

2. **Cutaneous Mycoses:** The fungi involving the skin, nails, and hair should be removed and examined directly under the microscope and cultured for the presence of organisms.

   a. Skin scrapings: The area of infection should be washed with 70% alcohol to remove surface contaminants. Scrapings should be taken from active border areas of the lesion and placed in a sterile container for laboratory study. Direct examination in 10% to 20% potassium hydroxide (KOH) is the most rapid method. Other methods including potassium hydroxide-glycerine, potassium hydroxide-ink, and the periodic acid-Schiff stain may be used. Cultures should be made for species identification.

In lesions that might contain *Candida albicans,* smears should be made on slides for staining and scrapings placed on Sabouraud agar for culture, as materials from lesions dry out rapidly if kept too long.

b. Nail scrapings: Scrapings or clippings of nails, especially near the bed of the nail, should be collected in a sterile container for examination. The same procedure is used as for skin except that the nail requires a longer period of time to clear in KOH even with gentle heating.

c. Hair: The basal portion of the hair or hair stubs should be plucked out with tweezers as the fungus usually is found in this part. The edges of the patches are likely to contain the best material. Wood's light (ultraviolet light rays of 3,660 angstrom units) under darkened conditions is useful in collecting infected hairs in scalp ringworm caused by most species of *Microsporum.* The infected hairs usually fluoresce with a bright yellowish-green color. Most species of *Trichophyton* and *M. gypseum* hair infections do not fluoresce. The hair may be placed in sterile paper containers, petri dishes, or on agar media and examined later in the laboratory.

3. **Subcutaneous Mycoses:** The diseases in this group include chromoblastomycosis, mycetoma (or maduromycosis), sporotrichosis, and rhinosporidiosis. The types of specimens from this group include: crusts and pus from open abscesses, exudate from lesions, aspirated fluids from unopened sinus tracts or abscesses, and tissue from biopsy. The organism, *Rhinosporidium seeberi,* causing rhinosporidiosis is difficult to culture at present, thus scrapings or biospy material should be examined directly or fixed for histological examination.

4. **Systemic Mycoses:** The deep or systemic mycoses may be diagnosed in the laboratory from pus or exudate, spinal fluid, sputum, bone marrow and blood, abscesses, and biopsies or autopsies. Direct examination, cultures, and in some cases animal inoculations should be made from material collected.

a. Pus or exudates: Specimens should be placed in sterile containers or as a drop on a slide with a cover glass placed over the material and pressed down to make a thin smear. A drop of 10% to 20% KOH may be added if clearing is necessary. Budding cells, large cells with endospores, or sulfur granules may be observed. Smears of pus should be stained by Gram method to see if branching hyphae, pseudomycelium, and budding forms are Gram-positive. Smears of the sulfur granule should be acid-fast stained. The specimens in the sterile containers should be cultured on media.

b. Spinal fluid: The fluid should be collected in a sterile container, centrifuged, and the sediment checked directly. If oval or budding cells are present, some of the sediment should be checked in India ink for capsule formation. Sediment should be stained by Gram method as well as by the acid-fast method in case actinomycetelike hyphae are evident. Cultures should be made.

c. Sputum: Sputum should be placed in a sterile container or smeared on a slide. The same procedure for examination as for pus should be followed. Gram method should be used to check for hyphae of actinomycetes, yeast cells of *Candida,* and arthrospores of *Geotrichum.* If there is blood in the sputum, a blood stain should be made and checked for *Histoplasma capsulatum.* An acid-fast stain will help indicate if *Nocardia* may be present.

If cryptococcosis is suspected, an India ink mount should be made. Cultures should be made either directly from the material taken from the patient or from the material in the sterile container.

TABLE I

Type of Specimen and Suggested Media for Isolation of the Fungi Causing Mycoses

DISEASE	CULTURE MEDIUM	TYPES OF SPECIMENS
Superficial Mycoses		
Tinea versicolor	None	Skin scrapings
Tinea nigra	Sabouraud + antibiotics[1]	Skin scrapings
Piedra	Sabouraud agar	Cut hair
Cutaneous Mycoses		
Tinea capitis	Sabouraud + antibiotics[1], or	Epilated hair
Tinea corporis, etc.	Dermatophyte Test Medium	Skin scrapings
Tinea unguium (Onychomycosis)		Nail scrapings
Candidiasis	Sabouraud + antibiotics[1] and Sabouraud agar	Skin scrapings Mucocutaneous scrapings Vaginal scrapings
Subcutaneous Mycoses		
Chromoblastomycosis	Sabouraud + antibiotics[1]	Scrapings, crust Exudate from lesion
Mycetoma (Maduromycosis)	Sabouraud agar Brain heart infusion agar BHI, blood agar	Pus from draining sinuses Aspirated fluids Biopsy material
Sporotrichosis	Sabouraud + antibiotics[1]	Pus from ulcerating lesions Aspirated fluid
Rhinosporidiosis	None	Biopsy of nasal or ocular polyps Skin scrapings
Systemic Mycosis		
(Actinomycetes)		
Actinomycosis	Brain-heart infusion agar BHI with 0.2% glucose Chopped meat medium (all anaerobic, 37° C)	Pus from draining sinuses Aspirated fluid Sputum, spinal fluid Bronchial washings
Nocardiosis	Sabouraud, BHI Blood agar (Incubate at room temp. and 37° C) Paraffin Bait Technique	Same as above
(Yeastlike fungi)		
Candidiasis	Sabouraud + antibiotics[1] Sabouraud agar (for species inhibited by antibiotics)	Sputum, bronchial washings Spinal fluid Urine, stools

(TABLE 1 cont.)

DISEASE	CULTURE MEDIUM	TYPES OF SPECIMENS

Cryptococcosis	Sabouraud + chloramphenicol
	Potato dextrose agar/urea-
	   antibiotics
	Creatinine medium
	   (at 24° and 37° C)
		Spinal fluid, sputum
		Pus from abscesses, sinus tracts
		Scrapings from skin lesions
		Urine

Geotrichosis	Sabouraud + chloramphenicol	Sputum, bronchial washings Stools
(Diphasic fungi)		

Blastomycosis
   North American
	Sabouraud + antibiotics[1]
	Brain-heart infusion agar
	   + antibiotics[1]
	BHI (no antibiotics) at 37° C
	   or Sabhi agar at 37° C
		Scrapings from edge of lesions
		Pus from abscesses, sinus tracts
		Urine, sputum
		Bronchial washings

Blastomycosis
   South American
	Same as above	Scrapings from edge of lesions
		Scrapings from mucous mem-
		   branes
		Biopsied lymph nodes
		Sputum, bronchial washings

Coccidioidomycosis	Sabouraud + antibiotics[1]	Sputum, bronchial washings Spinal fluid Urine Scrapings from lesions Pus from abscesses, sinuses

Histoplasmosis	BHI + antibiotics[1]
	Sabhi Blood agar/antibiotics
	BHI/6% blood at 37° C
	   or Sabhi Blood agar at
	   37° C
		Blood, bone marrow
		Sputum, bronchial washings
		Spinal fluid
		Pus from sinus tracts, or ulcers
		Skin scrapings from lesions

Miscellaneous Mycoses		
Aspergillosis	Sabouraud + chloramphenicol	Sputum, bronchial washings
Mucormycosis (Phycomycosis)	Sabouraud + chloramphenicol	Sputum, bronchial washings Biopsy material
Penicilliosis	Same as for Aspergillosis	Sputum, bronchial washings Nail scrapings
External Otitis (Otomycosis)	Sabouraud + chloramphenicol	Epithelial scales and detritus

[1]Antibiotics — include the addition of chloramphenicol and cycloheximide to the medium unless bacterial contamination is not likely. In such a case, chloramphenicol may be omitted.

d. <u>Bone marrow and blood</u>: Smears should be made of this material, stained with Giemsa or Wright stain, and examined for the presence of *H. capsulatum.* The specimen in the syringe should be expelled onto culture media in small quantities for streaking on the surface of the agar. If the bone marrow contains blood, larger quantities may be used (2-3 ml instead of 0.2-0.3 ml).

e. <u>Biopsies and Autopsies</u>: If the material is available from a biopsy or autopsy, make smears if direct examination is desirable, culture a portion, and prepare the remainder for histological sections.

NOTE: In handling of pathogenic fungi, routine precautions should be taken, including washing hands, use of sterile technique, disinfecting any contaminated surfaces with good fungicides, and sterilizing or burning all cultures or contaminated materials ready to be discarded.

Mailing of Specimens

Skin, nail, and hair placed in paper packets or envelopes may be mailed after enclosing them in regular envelopes. These specimens will usually arrive in viable condition.

Other specimens such as sputum, urine, exudates from lesions, etc., are usually of no value after shipment by mail as saprophytic fungi and bacteria multiply rapidly, reducing the chance of isolating the pathogenic fungus. In such cases the specimens from the patients should be put on media for culture whenever possible before the specimens are mailed.

For specific details on mailing and labeling of specimens the individual should consult the nearest state health departments or the local laboratories for specific requirements.

Selected References

1. AJELLO, L. 1951. Collecting specimens for the laboratory demonstration and isolation of fungi. J. Am. Med. Assoc. 146:1581.
2. AJELLO, L., L. K. Georg, W. Kaplan and L. Kaufman. 1963. Laboratory Manual for Medical Mycology. PHSP No. 994. Superintendent of Documents, U. S. Government Printing Office. Washington 25, D.C.
3. DVOŘAK, J. and M. Otčenašek. 1969. Mycological Diagnosis of Animal Dermatophytoses. Dr. W. Junk N. V., Publishers. The Hague.
4. EDWARDS, R. W. and E. Hartman. 1952. A simple technique for collecting fungus specimens from infected surfaces. Lloydia 15:39.
5. HALEY, L. D. 1964. Diagnostic Medical Mycology. Appleton-Century-Crofts. New York, N. Y.
6. MOSS, E. S. and A. L. McQuown. 1969. Atlas of Medical Mycology. The Williams and Wilkins Co. Baltimore.
7. ROBINSON, H. M., M. M. Cohen, R. C. V. Robinson and E. S. Berrston. 1956. Simplified office procedures for mycological diagnosis. J. Am. Med. Assoc. 160:537.
8. THOMPSON, A. N. 1955. Mycological teaching material. Am. J. Med. Tech. 21:57.

Cultivation of Fungi

The techniques used for cultivation of fungi are somewhat similar to those used by the medical bacteriologist. There are important differences to consider when handling fungi. A stiff nichrome wire needle (22 gauge) should be used for transferring cultures. A pair of dissecting needles is useful for teasing masses of mycelium apart on slides before mounting the material for better observation.

It is better to use test tubes or prescription bottles for culture of clinical specimens and for the study of cultures. Petri dishes are not recommended as these containers afford less protection from the more virulent organisms.

Medium: Sabouraud glucose agar with or without chloramphenicol and cycloheximide inhibitors will support most of the pathogenic forms for study. For some organisms specific media will be needed. Clinical specimens should be inoculated onto Sabouraud glucose agar with both antibiotics, chloramphenicol and cycloheximide. Modifications of the former medium under the name Mycosel or Mycobiotic agar are useful commercial media for this purpose. Mycophil agar with antibiotics is good for rapid isolation of pathogenic fungi. This same medium is good for maintenance of fungi. The Dermatophyte Test Medium is useful for skin, nail, or hair material.

Clinical material or a small portion from a known stock culture should be cut into the surface of the medium on the slant, using sterile technique at all times. The cultures should be incubated for one to two weeks and observed for colony formation.

When working with pathogenic fungi, the area should be wiped up with a fungicide such as 2% Amphyl or other similar antiseptics before and after a laboratory period or a wet paper towel may be kept below the area where the cultures are being handled.

Examination of Cultures

When cultures are grown on different media in slants, the characteristics of the fungus may be observed under the low power objective of the microscope by looking along the edges of the medium and colony.

1. Portions of colonies should be removed from the culture and placed on a slide with lactophenol cotton blue, teased apart, and covered with a cover glass for observation in the microscope. If spores or other structures are characteristic for identification of the fungus then no further procedures are necessary. The use of the cellophane tape-cover glass mount or the slide culture techniques will aid in determining the relationship of the spores. However, many organisms must be grown on special media, subjected to special physiological tests, or must be placed in animals for pathogenicity tests.

2. **Slide Culture:** In order to avoid disturbing the arrangement of the fungus structures, slide culture techniques can be utilized and permanently stained mounts made from the slide and cover glass. The following slide culture techniques may be of use for class or laboratory study of fungi:

    a. Riddell slide culture method: This involves growing the fungus on the sides of an agar block between a glass slide and cover glass in a moist chamber. For more details see procedure for culture of contaminants by this method, or the reference (Riddell, 1950). For additional methods see Littman (1949) and Taschdjian (1954).

3. **Cellophane Tape-cover Glass Mounts:** This method will keep more of the fungus structures intact than the direct mount method. See procedure under laboratory procedure for study of contaminant fungi.

Mounting Fluids and Staining Methods

Mounting Media

These media may be used for temporary mounts, and in some cases more permanent slide mounts.

1. **Potassium Hydroxide:** 10% to 20% solution. This method is one of the most rapid ones for direct examination of infected material. Gently heating the slide will increase the rate of clearing, and the fungus elements should be more readily observed. These specimens have been made permanent (Tasehdjian, 1955) by drawing off the alkaline mixture, neutralizing in 10% acetic acid, dehydrating in absolute alcohol, clearing in xylol, and mounting.

2. **Rapid Contrast Stain** (Swartz and Medrek, 1969): This method is useful for infected skin scales, nail scrapings, hairs, sputa, and pus with *Candida* sp. or other fungi. Preparation of stain:

    a. Modified KOH Solution.

    KOH 10%. . . . . 1 part

    Aerosol OTB 1%. . . . . 1 part

    Formula for OTB:
    Dioctyl sodium sulphosuccinate . . . . 0.85 g
    Sodium benzoate. . . . . 0.15 g/100 ml water

    Ink Blue PP 1% . . . . 2 parts

    This may be used for clearing infected skin, nails, and hairs to observe the fungus.

    b. Rose Bengal 0.5% in buffered Shear's mounting fluid.

    Preparation of Shear's mounting fluid:

    Potassium acetate 2% in pH 8 McIlvaine's buffer (0.2M)* . . . . 300 ml
    Glycerin . . . . 120 ml
    Ethyl alcohol 95% . . . . 180 ml
    *McIlvaine's buffer contains solution A (0.1M citric acid) and solution B (0.2M disodium hydrogen phosphate). Mix 0.55 ml of solution A with 19.45 ml of solution B.

    Mix one part of a with 2 parts of b and add 0.83% KOH, 0.17% Ink Blue PP, and 0.083% aerosol OTB to make up for the dilution of b. Place a drop of the contrast stain on a slide, add infected material, cover slip, heat gently until bubbles appear. The fungal elements are stained light blue and the background material is rose-red.

3. **Fountain Pen Ink and Potassium Hydroxide:** A mixture of 9 parts potassium hydroxide (10%) and 1 part blue-black ink is useful for scrapings containing such fungi as *Malassezia furfur* and *Candida albicans.*

4. **KOH and DMSO Medium** (Azias and Taplin, 1966). Useful to demonstrate fungi in skin, nail, or hair scrapings after 1 minute without heat. Not recommended if more than 20 minutes elapse before examination of material in the preparation. The medium contains 20% KOH by weight in a solution of 60% water and 40% DMSO (dimethyl sulfoxide).

5. **Potassium Hydroxide and Glycerin:** Pus and sputum can be maintained for a longer period of time by placing in an aqueous solution containing 5% potassium hydroxide and 25% glycerin.

6. **Lactophenol cotton blue** (Aman's medium): This is an excellent medium for mounting most fungi:

    Lactic acid . . . . 20 g
    Phenol crystals . . . . 20 g

Glycerin . . . . 40 g

Water . . . . 20 ml

The 0.05 g of cotton blue (add after solution completed) may be added to make the hyaline fungal structures more distinct.

7. **India Ink:** A drop of India ink is placed on a glass slide with a loopful of the *Cryptococcus neoformans* culture and stirred together. A cover glass is added quickly and examined for capsules, which are readily demonstrated by this method. If the India ink is too dark, it may be diluted.

8. **Mounting Medium for Permanent Preparations** (Koch, 1963): The medium consists of 10 g polyvinyl alcohol (intermediate viscosity), 20 g chloral hydrate, 35 ml lactic acid, 25 ml 15% phenol, 10 ml glycerin, and 50 ml distilled water. Store in a tightly closed dark bottle. Material that has been stained in lactophenol cotton blue, or from KOH solution, may be maintained in the medium without loss of color in most cases. To prevent excess drying, the cover glass may be sealed.

9. **Direct Staining on Vinyl Plastic Tape** (Keddie, et al., 1961): Scotch brand tapes #681 and #473 are recommended for use in stripping and staining for fungal infection of the horny epidermis. Place tape with material, adhesive side up, on a slide and stain 1 minute with Hucker crystal violet, Loeffler methylene blue, or Giemsa solution. Rinse with alcohol for a moment, dry and mount in permanent or temporary mounting media.

10. **Other Mounting Media:** A number of other media for mounting fungi may be found in references.

11. **Nail Polish, Laktoseal,*** or other materials may be used to seal the lactophenol, glycerin, or mounting media on slides.

Staining Methods

1. **Periodic Acid-Schiff Stain:** An excellent stain for differentiating fungi in scrapings and tissue sections.

    a. <u>For skin scrapings</u>: Spread thin scrapings on a slide coated with Mayer's albumen. The scrapings may be collected directly with the fixative placed on the lesion. Scrape the surface scales off and immediately press them on the surface of a clean slide. Heat gently and check to see if skin scrapings are fast on slide before proceeding.

    Use 3 or 4 drops to cover or immerse the fixed scrapings:

    (1) Immerse 1 minute in 95% alcohol.

    (2) Immerse in 5% periodic acid 5 minutes.

    (3) Immerse in the following solution for 2 minutes:

    Basic fuchsin . . . . 0.1 g

    95% alcohol . . . . 5.0 ml

    Water . . . . 95.0 ml

    (4) Rinse in tap water.

    (5) Immerse for 10 minutes in the following solution:

    Zinc (or sodium) hydrosulfite . . . . 1.0 g

    Tartaric acid . . . . 0.5 g

    Water . . . . 100.0 ml

*ESBE Laboratory Supplies, 3431 Bathurst St., Toronto 19, Ontario, Canada.

(6) Rinse in tap water.

(7) Counterstain with <u>one</u> of the following:

Saturated aqueous solution of picric acid for two minutes, or light green for 5 seconds:

Light green.................................... 1.0 g

Glacial acetic acid.............................. 0.25 ml

80% alcohol ....100.0 ml

(8) Rinse for a short time in tap water.

(9) Dehydrate about 10 seconds in 95% alcohol, 1 minute in 100% alcohol, rinse twice in xylol for about 1 minute each and mount in permount or other mounting media.

The fungi stain a bright red or purplish-red after periodic acid hydrolysis to release aldehydes which can combine with Schiff reagent. The carbohydrates in the cell wall will take the red stain as a result of the reaction.

b. <u>For Tissue Sections</u>: Tissues should be fixed, dehydrated, embedded in paraffin, and sectioned by the routine method:

(1) Place in xylol to deparaffinize.

(2) Rinse in 100% alcohol.

(3) Wash in distilled water.

(4) Immerse in 1% periodic acid for 10 minutes.

(5) Rinse in tap water 5-10 minutes.

(6) Immerse in the following solution for 2 minutes:

Basic fuchsin.................................... 0.1 g

95% alcohol .... 5.0 ml

Water ....95.0 ml

(7) Rinse in tap water for 30 seconds.

(8) Immerse for 30 minutes (or possibly up to 2-3 hours for some material) in the following:

Zinc (or sodium) hydrosulfite .... 1.0 g

Tartaric acid.................................... 0.5 g

Water ....100.0 ml

(9) Rinse in tap water 3-5 minutes.

(10) Immerse in light green for 2 minutes:

Light green.................................... 1.0 g

Glacial acetic acid .... 0.25 ml

80% alcohol ....100.0 ml

(11) Rinse for a short time in tap water.

(12) Dehydrate about 10 seconds in 95% alcohol, 1 minute in 100% alcohol, rinse twice in xylol for about 1 minute each and mount in permount or other mounting media.

NOTE: Hematoxylin and eosin stained slides may be restained by removal of the cover glass with xylol and rehydration. The slide is then placed in 1% periodic acid for ten minutes and the rest of the procedure is continued. This technique is useful when the hematoxylin and eosin stain does not differentiate the fungus from the tissue sufficiently well.

2. **Gram's Method (Hucker Modification):** All fungi are Gram-positive when stained by the Gram method.

   a. Procedure:

     (1) Fix the smear.

     (2) Place crystal violet on slide - 1 minute.

     (3) Wash.

     (4) Apply Gram's iodine solution - 1 minute.

     (5) Wash.

     (6) Decolorize in 95% alcohol (or equal parts of alcohol and acetone).

     (7) Counterstain Safranin for 10 seconds.

     (8) Wash and dry.

   b. Reagents:

     (1) Ammonium oxalate-crystal violet solution:

       Crystal violet (85% dye content) . . . . 4 g

       Ethyl alcohol (95%) . . . . 20 ml

      Dissolve the dye in the alcohol; dilute solution 1:10 with distilled water.

       Ammonium oxalate . . . . 0.8 g

       Water . . . . 80.0 ml

      Dissolve the ammonium oxalate in water. Mix 1 part of the crystal violet solution with 4 parts of ammonium oxalate solution.

     (2) Gram's iodine solution:

       Iodine . . . . 1 g

       Potassium iodide . . . . 2 g

      Dissolve in 5 ml of distilled water, then make-up to 240 ml with water. Add 60 ml of a 5% solution of sodium bicarbonate.

     (3) Counterstain:

       Safranin (2.5% solution in 95% alcohol) . . . . 10 ml

       Water . . . . 100 ml

3. **Acid-fast Stain (Kinyoun's Modification):** This stain is especially useful as an aid in differentiation of *Nocardia* sp. The hyphae of *N. asteroides* and *N. brasiliensis* will appear partially acid-fast or acid-fast. Acid-fast organism stain red.

   a. Procedure:

     (1) Make smear and heat-fix.

     (2) Kinyoun carbol fuchsin is applied over smear. Stain at room temperature for 3 minutes.

     (3) Wash. Decolorize for 5 to 10 seconds with acid alcohol (no more).

     (4) Wash in water.

     (5) Counterstain ½ minute with methylene blue.

     (6) Rinse quickly with water; dry, and examine under oil.

   b. Reagents:

     (1) Kinyoun carbol fuchsin:

       Basic fuchsin . . . . 4.0 g

       Phenol . . . . 8.0 g

Alcohol (95%) . . . . 20.0 ml

Water (distilled) . . . . 100.0 ml

(2) Acid alcohol:

Hydrochloric acid, Concentrated . . . .   3 ml

Ethyl alcohol, 95% . . . .   97 ml

(3) Methylene blue:

Methylene blue . . . .   2.5 g

Alcohol (95%) . . . . 100.0 g

4. **Giemsa Stain:** This stain and others — Gridley, periodic acid-Schiff, or Gomori-silver-methenamine are useful to locate *Histoplasma capsulatum* in the reticuloendothelial cells.

a. Procedure:

(1) Fix the smear with 100% methyl alcohol for about 3 to 5 minutes.

(2) Add mixed staining solution; leave for about 15 minutes.

(3) Wash well in tap water.

(4) Dry by blotting with bibulous paper.

b. Reagents:

(1) Stain solution (stock):

Giemsa powder . . . . 600.0 mg

Methyl alcohol (acetone-free) . . . . 50.0 ml

Glycerin (neutral, freshly opened supply) . . . . 50.0 ml

Grind the powder in a mortar and weigh. Then place it in the mortar again with a portion of the glycerin, and regrind. Pour the upper one-third into a chemically clean flask, add more glycerin, and regrind. Add stopper to flask and place in water bath at 55° C. for 2 hours. Shake every ½ hour (lightly). Use a part of the alcohol to wash out the mortar. Remove the mixture from the bath at the end of 2 hours, cool, and add alcohol washings from mortar. After stain has ripened for about 2 weeks, it is ready for use. The undissolved portion can be filtered or may settle out. The solution can be placed in a dropper bottle.

(2) Buffer solution (pH 7.2):

Na_2HPO_4 (anhydrous) . . . .   6.77 g

KH_2PO_4 . . . .   2.59 g

Distilled water to . . . . 1000.00 ml

(3) Staining solution:

Stain solution (stock) . . . .   2 ml

Buffer solution . . . .   6 ml

Mix well before using.

5. **Acridine Orange Stain:** See procedure under tinea versicolor (page 58).

6. **Other Staining Methods:** Additional staining techniques including Gomori methenamine-silver nitrate technique, Gridley histological stain, and others may be found in various references and textbooks.

7. **Fluorescent Antibody Technique for Fungi:** Currently the FA technique is being used on a limited scale in some mycology laboratories. An excellent summary of the current status and the procedures are given in the *Laboratory Manual for Medical Mycology* by Ajello, Georg,

Kaplan and Kaufman (1963), and in the *Laboratory Identification of Pathogenic Fungi Simplified* by Hazen, Gordon, and Reed (1970). Until a better evaluation of the techniques have been made by a number of technicians and the specific conjugates for fungi are available commercially, the procedures will continue to be used on a limited basis in the laboratories.

Selected References

1. AJELLO, L., L. K. Georg, W. Kaplan and L. Kaufman. 1963. Laboratory Manual for Medical Mycology. PHSP No. 994. Superintendent of Documents, U. S. Government Printing Office. Washington, D.C. 20402.

2. BROWN, J. H. and L. Brenn. 1931. Methods for differentiational staining of Gram-positive and Gram-negative bacteria in tissue sections. Bull. Johns Hopkins Hosp. 48:69.

3. CHICK, E. W. 1961. Acridine orange fluorescent stain for fungi. Archs. Derm. 83(2):305.

4. COHEN, M. M. 1954. A simple procedure for staining tinea versicolor with fountain pen ink. J. Invest. Derm. 22:9.

5. EMMONS, C. W., C. H. Binford and J. P. Utz. 1963. Medical Mycology. Appendix III. pp. 354. Histopathologic procedures and special stains for fungi. Lea and Febiger, Philadelphia, Pa.

6. GORDON, M. A. 1951. Rapid permanent staining and mounting of skin scraping and hair. Arch. Derm. and Syph. 63:343.

7. GRIDLEY, M. F. 1953. A stain for fungi in tissue sections. Am. J. Clin. Path. 23:303.

8. GROCOTT, R. G. 1955. Technical Bulletin of the Registry of Medical Technologists, Am. J. Clin. Path. 25(7):975.

9. HAZEN, E. S., M. A. Gordon, and F. C. Reed. 1970. Laboratory Identification of Pathogenic Fungi Simplified. 3rd Edition. Charles C. Thomas. Springfield, Ill.

10. KAPLAN, W. and L. Kaufman. 1961. The application of fluorescent antibody techniques to medical mycology – a review. Sabouraudia 1(3):137.

11. KEDDIE, F., A. Orr and D. Liebes. 1961. Direct staining on vinyl plastic tape, demonstration of the cutaneous flora of the epidermis by the strip method. Sabouraudia 1(2):108.

12. KLIGMAN, A. M. and H. Mescon. 1950. The periodic acid-Schiff stain for demonstration of fungi in animal tissues. J. Bact. 60:415.

13. KOCH, H. A. 1963. Ein neues Einschluss medium für mykologische Dauerpräparate. Mykosen. 6(2):27.

14. KRAMER, J. and A. Kirshbaum. 1960. Cylinder plate assays for amphotericin B in dosage forms and body fluids. Antibiot. and Chemother. 10(3):188.

15. LITTMAN, M. L. 1949. Improved slide culture technique for study and identification of pathogenic fungi. Am. J. Clin. Path. 19:278.

16. MALLORY, F. B. 1942. Pathological Technique. W. B. Saunders Co. Philadelphia, Pa.

17. PADHYE, A. A. 1969. Cellophane mounts of ascigerous states of dermatophytes and other keratinophilic fungi. Mycologia 60:1242.

18. PEABODY, J. W. 1955. Demonstration of fungi by periodic acid-Schiff stain in pulmonary granuloma. J. Am. Med. Assoc. 157:8858.

19. REYNOLDS, R. C., L. Stinson and B. Hatten. 1964. Plastic tissue-culture dishes in diagnostic mycology. Am. J. Clin. Path. 41:385.

20. RIDDELL, R. W. 1950. Permanent stained mycological preparations obtained by slide culture. Mycologia 42:265.

21. SHARVILL, D. 1952. The periodic acid-Schiff stain in the diagnosis of dermatomycosis. Brit. J. Derm. 64:329.

22. SWARTZ, J. H. and T. F. Medrek. 1969. Rapid contrast stain as a diagnostic aid for fungus infections. Archs. Derm. 99:494.

23. TASCHDJIAN, C. L. 1954. Simplified technique for growing fungi in slide culture. Mycologia 46:681.

24. TUITE, J. 1969. Plant Pathological Methods. Fungi and Bacteria. Burgess Publishing Co., Minneapolis, Minn.

25. ZAIAS, N. and D. Taplin. 1966. Improved preparation for the diagnosis of mycologic diseases. Archs. Derm. 93:608.

Media

All materials considered possible cases of mycotic infections should be cultured even though the direct examination of the material failed to reveal the presence of a fungus. Routinely, isolations from the specimens should be made on the specified media and incubated at 37° C and at 24° C if the source is from a subcutaneous or systemic type infection. Skin, nail, or hair from cases of dermatomycoses are usually isolated on Sabouraud glucose agar slants or plates with the addition of cycloheximide and chloramphenicol, or on the dermatophyte test medium at 24° C.

Media for General Use

Media can be obtained commercially in dehydrated form. Addition of antibiotics is desirable in some cases.

1. **Blood Agar Base** (commercially prepared): This medium with the addition of 10 mg of thiamine per liter may aid in macroconidial production at room temperature in *Trichophyton mentagrophytes, T. rubrum, T. schoenleinii, T. verrucosum,* and *T. violaceum.*

2. **Brain-heart-infusion Blood Agar** (commercially prepared): for isolating and maintaining the yeast phase of some of the systemic fungi, with or without blood, at 37° C. Also for growth of *Actinomyces* sp.

3. **Brain-heart-infusion Agar with Cycloheximide* and Chloramphenicol:**** This medium is for primary isolation of *Histoplasma capsulatum* and *Blastomyces dermatitidis* at room temperature (24-25° C). At 37° C the yeast phases of dimorphic fungi should be grown without cycloheximide in the medium.

   Formula:

Brain-heart infusion	37 g
Cycloheximide	0.5 g
Chloramphenicol	0.05 g
Agar	20 g
Distilled water	1000 ml

4. **Cornmeal Agar:** This medium when prepared in the laboratory from cornmeal can be used to stimulate chlamydospore production in *Candida albicans.* The addition of 1% glucose to the agar can be used to differentiate *Trichophyton rubrum* and *T. mentagrophytes,* based on pigment formation. This medium is useful in stimulating sporulation of many fungi, and for slide culture studies. (Commercially available.)

   a. Procedure:

Cornmeal	40 g
Water	1000 ml
Agar	20 g

   Simmer cornmeal and water for one hour. Filter or decant, bring volume up to 1000 ml and add agar; melt and filter again if necessary. Autoclave.

5. **Czapek's Agar:** Especially useful in the study of the colony characteristics of *Nocardia* sp., *Penicillium* sp., and *Aspergillus* sp.

---

*Actidione (The Upjohn Co., Kalamazoo, Mich.)
**Chloromycetin (Parke-Davis and Co., Detroit, Mich.)

<u>Formula</u>:

Sucrose	30 g
Sodium nitrate	3 g
Dipotassium phosphate	1 g
Magnesium sulfate	0.5 g
Potassium chloride	0.5 g
Ferrous sulfate	0.01 g
Water	1000 ml
Agar	15 g

6. **Potato Dextrose Agar** (commercially available): This medium is useful for spore production.

Peeled, diced potatoes, infusion from	200 g
Glucose	20 g
Agar	15 g (or 20 g)
Distilled water	1000 ml

Preparation as for cornmeal if infusion is made. The use of 2% agar insures a drier surface on the agar medium

7. **Mycophil Agar:** For cultivation and maintenance of fungi, isolation of *Streptomyces;* with the addition of antibiotics is similar to Mycosel (a BBL BioQuest product).* Composition:

Phytone peptone	10 g
Glucose	10 g
Agar	16 g
Distilled water	1000 ml

8. **Sabouraud-cycloheximide-chloramphenicol Agar** (Mycobiotic Agar, Difco).**

<u>Formula</u>:

Sabouraud glucose agar plus 5 grams of agar (2% agar content) per liter	65.0 g
Cycloheximide***	0.5 g
Chloramphenicol****	0.05 g
Distilled water	1000.0 ml

Add the 65 g of dehydrated Sabouraud glucose agar to 1000 ml of distilled water and heat to boiling. Add and mix 0.05 g of chloramphenicol which has been suspended and heated quickly in 10 ml of 95% alcohol. Add the cycloheximide in a 10 ml acetone solution to the medium and mix well, tube, and autoclave for 10 minutes.

This medium is useful for isolation of pathogenic fungi from clinical materials heavily contaminated with bacteria and saprophytic fungi. Some of the organisms inhibited or partially inhibited by cycloheximide are: *Cryptococcus neoformans, Trichosporon beigelii, Allescheria boydii, Aspergillus fumigatus, Candida krusei, C. tropicalis, C. parapsilosis,* and *Nocardia asteroides.*

9. **Sabouraud Glucose Agar:** For primary isolation and maintenance of cultures (commercially available).

*Bioquest, Cockeysville, Md.
**Difco Laboratories, Inc., Detroit, Mich.
***Actidione (The Upjohn Co., Kalamazoo, Mich.)
****Chloromycetin (Parke-Davis and Co., Detroit, Mich.)

Formula:

Glucose	40 g
Neopeptone	10 g
Agar	15 g
Water	1000 ml

Adjust pH to 5.6.

The addition of 10 mg of thiamine per liter enhances the growth of some of the dermatophytes, especially *T. verrucosum.* If the dehydrated product is used or the medium is used for slide cultures, 2% agar should be used to insure a firm dry surface.

Media for Specific Use
(Many are prepared commercially.)

The following media have been developed for growth of specific pathogenic fungi as routine isolation media are not always suitable.

A. *Actinomyces* **species**

1. **Casitone Starch Agar:** This medium is used to indicate if the organism hydrolyzes starch under anaerobic conditions as indicated by the Gram iodine reaction on the surface of the culture.

   Formula:

Heart infusion broth (Difco)	25 g
Casitone (Difco)	4 g
Yeast extract	5 g
Soluble starch	5 g
Agar	15 g
Distilled water	1000 ml

   Dissolve the components, adjust the pH to 7.0 and dispense 8 ml in tubes.

2. **Howell and Pines Casitone Medium:**

Casitone (Difco)	15.00 g
Yeast extract	5.00 g
Glucose (anhydrous)	5.00 g
NaCl	2.50 g
L-cysteine hydrochloride	0.75 g
K_2HPO_4	1.20 g
KH_2PO_4	1.20 g
Disodium ethylene diamine tetra-acetic acid	0.25 g
Agar	0.75 g
Distilled water up to	1000.00 ml

   Adjust pH to 7.3.

   Add agar to 200 ml of water and autoclave. Sterilize the rest of the constituents by Seitz filtration and add the cooled agar solution aseptically.

3. **Thioglycollate Medium:** For primary isolation of *Actinomyces* species.

   Formula:

Tryptocase	20 g
NaCl	5 g
Dipotassium phosphate	2 g
Sodium thioglycollate	1 g
Methylene blue	0.002 g
Agar	0.5 g
Water	1000 ml

4. **Gelatin.** Liquefaction. For actinomycetes.

   Formula:

Gelatin	100 g
Heart infusion Broth (Difco)	25 g
Casitone (Difco)	4 g
Glucose	5 g
Yeast Extract	5 g
Distilled water	1000 ml

   Dissolve, adjust the pH to 7.0 and tube. Add cotton plugs and autoclave. Use pyrogallol-carbonate seal, incubate 4 weeks at 37° C.

   Preparation of pyrogallol-carbonate seals. Cut off top of cotton plug leaving sufficient space so a small amount of absorbent cotton can be added to extend down about ½ inch from the top of tube. Add 5 drops of pyrogallol solution and 5 drops of 10% Na_2CO_2 solution, then insert a rubber stopper. (The pyrogallol solution contains 100 g of pyrogallic acid plus 150 ml of water.)

5. **Litmus Milk.** Medium for actinomycetes, etc.

   Formula:

Skim milk powder	100 g
Litmus	750 mg
Yeast Extract	5 g
Glucose	3 g
Distilled water	1000 ml

   The medium is dissolved, the pH adjusted to 7, tubed and autoclaved at 10 lbs. pressure. Inoculate, then add the pyrogallol-carbonate seals on cotton plugs, incubate for 4 weeks at 37° C.

6. **Nitrate Reduction.** Medium for actinomycetes.

   Formula:

Heart Infusion Broth (Difco)	25 g
Yeast extract	5 g
Casitone (Difco)	4 g
KNO_3	1 g
Distilled water	1000 ml

Dissolve, adjust pH to 7, tube, cotton-plug, and autoclave. Add pyrogallol-carbonate seals and incubate at 37° C. Test small amounts 2 or 3 times during a two-week interval for nitrite reaction (a few drops of both sulfanilic acid solution* and dimethyl-alpha-naphthylamine solution**), which should show a red to brown color, if nitrates are reduced to nitrites. Zinc may be used to reduce the remaining nitrates or to see if the organism did not reduce nitrates.

7. **Sugar Fermentations.** Especially for actinomycetes.

   Formula:

Heart infusion broth (Difco)	25 g
Yeast extract	5 g
Casitone (Difco)	4 g
Brome cresol purple (0.04%)	15 ml
Distilled water	1000 ml

Dissolve, adjust pH to 7, tube, and autoclave. Add sterile sugars to make a final concentration of 0.5%.

Transfer the organism to the fermentation tubes and seal with pyrogallol-carbonate seals. Incubate for 1 month at 37° C, checking for acid and gas formation periodically.

8. **Actinomyces Maintenance Medium** (Pine and Watson, 1959).

   Formula: Semi-Solid Medium

   Part I (Salts Solution)

KH_2PO_4	60 g
$(NH_4)_2SO_4$	4 g
$MgSO_4 \cdot 7H_2O$	0.8 g
$CaCl_2$	0.08 g
Distilled water	500 ml

Adjust pH to 7.2 with 20% KOH, and dilute to 1000 ml with distilled water.

   Part II

Heart infusion broth (Difco)	25 g
Glucose	5 g
Cysteine HCl	1 g
Casitone (Difco)	4 g
Yeast extract	5 g
Soluble starch	1 g
Agar	7 g
Distilled water	750 ml

Combine 250 ml of the salts solution (Part I) with 750 ml of Part II. Adjust pH to 7.2. Dispense 8 ml per tube and plug (cotton). Autoclave for 10 minutes at 15 lbs (120° C). Final pH 6.8-7.0. For solid medium use 20 g of agar instead of 7 g or no agar for liquid medium.

---

*Sulfanilic Acid Solution: Glacial acetic acid, 100 ml.; water, 250 ml.: sulfanilic acid, 2.8g.
**Dimethyl-alpha-naphthylamine solution: Glacial acetic acid, 100 ml.; water, 250 ml.; dimethyl-alpha-naphthylamine, 2.1 ml.

B. Antigens — media for preparation of coccidioidin, histoplasmin broth:

Formula:

L-asparagine	7.00 g
Ammonium chloride	7.00 g
K_2HPO_4 (anhydrous)	1.31 g
$Na_3C_6H_5O_7\,5\frac{1}{2}H_2O$, c.p.	0.90 g
$MgSO_4 \cdot 7H_2O$ (U.S.P.)	1.50 g
Ferric citrate (U.S.P.)	0.30 g
Glucose (U.S.P.)	10.00 g
Glycerine, c.p. (U.S.P.)	25.00 g
Distilled water up to	1000.00 ml

Dissolve asparagine in 300 ml of hot water (50° C). Use 25 ml of water to dissolve each of the organic salts, applying heat for ferric citrate. Add each salt in order to the warm asparagine solution (50° C) beginning with K_2HPO_4. Mix well, and add the remaining constituents. If 1500 ml quantities are used in Fernbach culture flask, sterilize at 115° C for 25 min.

C. *Candida* species:

1. **Beef Extract Broth:** For use in carbohydrate fermentation tests.

   Formula:

Beef extract	3.0 g
Peptone	10.0 g
NaCl	5.0 g
Distilled water	1000.0 ml
Bromcresol purple, stock solution	1.0 ml

   Heat to dissolve, adjust pH to 7.2, tube in 9 ml quantities, and sterilize at 120° C for 15 min.

   Bromcresol purple solution for stock:

Bromcresol purple	1.6 g
Alcohol, 95%	100.0 ml

   Stock carbohydrate solutions:

   10% aqueous solutions for dextrose, maltose, sucrose, and lactose, sterilized.

   Add 1 ml of one of the carbohydrates to one tube containing 9 ml of sterile beef extract broth.

2. **Chlamydospore Agar:** This is a commercially prepared medium that is good for chlamydospore formation.

3. **Cornmeal-Tween 80 Agar:** See procedure under cornmeal. Add 10 g of Tween 80 to the medium to enhance chlamydospore formation.

4. **Rice Agar with Tween 80** (commercially available): For chlamydospore formation (Taschdjian, 1957).

   Formula:

Cream of Rice	10 g
Tap water	1000 ml

Agar . . . . 10 g

Tween 80 . . . . 10 g

Add Cream of Rice to boiling water, and boil for ½ minute, filter, make up to 1000 ml, add agar and Tween 80, and sterilize.

5. **Serum Tube Method:** For production of germ tubes (Taschdjian et al., 1960).

Procedure:

Inoculate 0.5 ml of serum in a small tube with the organism.

Incubate at 37° C for 2 to 3 hours.

Check for germ tubes or short filamentous outgrowths from the oval or rounded cells of *Candida albicans*. The germ tubes are characteristic of this species.

Serum: Fresh or inactivated human serum and deep-frozen stored serum are satisfactory, as well as rabbit, guinea pig, horse, and bovine sera. Heat-coagulated serum is not satisfactory.

D. *Nocardia* **species:**

1. **Casein Medium:** For differentiation of *Nocardia* and *Streptomyces* species.

Formula:

Solution a.

Skim milk (dehydrated, or instant nonfat) . . . . 10 g

Distilled water . . . . 100 ml

Solution b.

Distilled water . . . . 100 ml

Agar . . . . 2 g

Autoclave both solutions separately, cool, and mix together. Pour into petri dishes.

2. **Gelatin Liquefaction Medium:** For aerobic actinomycetes.

Formula:

Nutrient broth . . . . 8 g

Gelatin . . . . 120 g

Demineralized water . . . . 1 liter

Autoclave at 121° C for 12 min. Inoculate the organisms slightly below the surface and incubate at 24° or 37° C along with a control. After growth occurs, refrigerate until control solidifies and check results.

3. **Paraffin Bait Technique** (Mishra and Randhawa, 1969): Clinical specimens with *Nocardia asteroides* may be isolated by application of the paraffin bait technique. This organism has been repeatedly isolated from soil by this method (McClung, 1960).

Procedure:

Homogenize sputa or gastric washings by shaking with glass beads. Mix 2 ml of the homogenized specimen with 5 ml of sterile carbon-free broth, put in a sterile test tube, and introduce a paraffin-coated glass rod (previously immersed for 10-12 hours in 95% alcohol) after the alcohol has drained off. Incubate at 37° C. Check growth after 1, 2, 4, and 6 weeks.

Carbon-free broth Formula:

$NaNO_3$	2.0 g
K_2HPO_4	0.8 g
$MgSO_4 \cdot 7H_2O$	0.5 g
$FeCl_3$	10.0 mg
$MnCl_2 \cdot 4H_2O$	8.0 mg
$ZnSO_4$	2.0 mg
Distilled water	1000.0 ml

Adjust pH to 7.0.

E. *Cryptococcus Neoformans* — **selective media.**

1. **Selective Isolation Medium** (Shields and Ajello, 1966): Colonies of *Cryptococcus neoformans* produce a brown pigment at 24 or 37° C. Other species of *Cryptococcus* and *Candida* grow on this medium without pigment production.

Formula:

Glucose	10.0 g
Creatinine	780.0 mg
Chloramphenicol	50.0 mg
Diphenyl (dissolved in 10 ml of 95% ethanol)	100.0 mg
Guizotia abyssinica (thistle) extract	200.0 ml
Distilled water	800.0 ml
Agar	20.0 g

The medium is prepared in the usual way. Plates or test tubes may be used for species differentiation.

2. **Tyrosine or Xanthine Agar.** For aerobic actinomycetes.

Formula:

Nutrient agar	23 g
Tyrosine	5 g
or	
(Xanthine	4 g)
Demineralized water	1 liter

Dissolve the nutrient agar in 500 ml of water and add either tyrosine or xanthine and mix. Make up to 1 liter and distribute crystals evenly. Adjust to pH 7.0. Autoclave for 15 minutes at 121 C. Pour into plates with crystals distributed evenly in the medium.

3. **Potato Dextrose Urea Medium** (Vogel, 1969): This is a selective medium for isolation of *Cryptococcus* and *Candida* species.

Formula:

Potato dextrose agar (commercial)	1000 ml
Urea agar base (filter-sterilized) (commercial)	100 ml

Adjust pH to 3.5 by addition of about 35 ml of 0.5N HCl to 1 liter of medium (Yellow).

Add a concentration of 100 units/ml of chloramphenicol before dispensing into dishes.

While the potato dextrose agar is still hot after sterilization, the urea agar base is added and the pH is adjusted. Saprophytic fungi can be inhibited by the addition of diphenyl at a concentration of 0.01%. At 37° C most *Cryptococcus* species will not grow. A red halo develops around *C. neoformans* from the breakdown of urea.

F. *Trichophyton, Microsporum* **species. Special media.**

1. **Agar Medium for Ascigerous State** (Weitzman and Silva-Hutner, 1967): This medium serves as a nonkeratinous soil-free substrate for production of cleistothecia by species of *Nannizzia* and *Arthroderma*.

   Formula:

$MgSO_4 \cdot 7H_2O$	1 g
KH_2PO_4	1 g
$NaNO_3$	1 g
Hunt's tomato paste	10 g
Beechnut baby oatmeal	10 g
Agar	18 g
Distilled water	1000 ml

   Adjust pH to 5.6 with NaOH.

   Autoclave at 121° C for 20 min.

2. **Modified Hair-Bait Technique** (Orr, 1969): The addition of Actidione with penicillin and streptomycin to sterile distilled water in the hair-bait technique increases the number of keratinophilic fungi recovered from soil samples.

   Procedure:

   Soil is placed in sterile petri plates containing 3 x 9 cm filter discs to aid in maintaining moisture. The soil is moistened with sterile distilled water containing 500 mg penicillin, 300 mg streptomycin and 0.5 mg Actidione/ml. The soil is baited with human or horse hair (sterilized).

   Check hair periodically for about 1 month, and identify if possible or place hair with fungal growth on media with cycloheximide and chloramphenicol. Later identify colonies.

3. **Dermatophyte Test Medium**[1] (DTM) (Taplin, et al, 1969): This is a color indicator medium for dermatophytes. Most of the dermatophytes produce a red color in the medium while most saprophytic fungi, yeasts, and bacteria do not modify the yellow color.

   Formula:

Phytone	10 g*
Glucose	10 g
Agar	20 g
Phenol red solution	40 ml
HCl, 0.8 M	6 ml
Cycloheximide	0.5 g**
Gentamicin sulfate	100 μ/ml***
Chlortetracycline HCl	100 μ/ml****

[1]Dermatophyte Test Medium (DTM): Commercially available, Chas. Pfizer & Co., Diagnostics Division, 300 W. 43rd St., New York, N.Y. 10036.
*Bioquest, Cockeysville, Md.
**The Upjohn Company, Kalamazoo, Mich.
***Schering Corp., Bloomfield, N.J.
****Lederle Laboratories, Div. of American Cyanamid Co., Pearl River, N. Y.

<u>Preparation:</u>

Ingredients must be obtained from sources indicated. Substitution of other brands changes the specificity and effectiveness of the medium.

1. Add the phytone, dextrose, and agar to 1,000 ml distilled water and boil to dissolve the agar.

2. Add 40 ml of phenol red solution while stirring. (Phenol red solution: 0.5 g Difco Bacto-phenol red dissolved in 15 ml 0.1 N NaOH made up to 100 ml with glass distilled water.)

3. Adjust pH of medium with 6 ml 0.8 M HCl added while stirring.

4. Dissolve 0.5 g cycloheximide in 2 ml acetone and add to hot medium while stirring.

5. Dissolve gentamicin sulfate in 2 ml glass distilled water and add to medium while stirring.

6. Autoclave at 12 lb pressure for ten minutes and cool to approximately 47° C.

7. Dissolve chlortetracycline in 25 ml sterile glass distilled water in sterile flask. Add to medium while stirring.

8. Dispense 8 ml amounts in sterile 1-oz screw cap bottles, slant, and cool. The final pH is about 5.5 and should be yellow in color.

9. For maximum shelf life, store in refrigerator.

Microscopic features must be checked for positive identification although a nonmycologist can now recognize most dermatophytes by the red color change in the colony. If there is bacterial or soil contamination on the skin or nails, the surface must be cleaned first or the medium loses its value as too many contaminants increase the number of false positives. The false positives may be some of the saprophytic fungi, yeasts, and bacteria. Cultures should be incubated at 22° to 30° C with the caps loose for up to 14 days before evaluating the color change from yellow to red for the dermatophytes.

4. **Medium for** *Trichophyton* **Species Identification*** (Georg and Camp, 1957):

a. <u>Casein agar base</u> (commercially available):

<u>Formula:</u>

Casamino acid (Difco), vitamin-free	2.5 g
Glucose	40.0 g
MgSO$_4$	0.1 g
KH$_2$PO$_4$	1.8 g
Agar	20.0 g
Distilled water up to	1000.0 g

Adjust pH to 6.8. Heat to dissolve ingredients, tube, or put in flasks and sterilize.

b. <u>Casein agar base plus inositol</u> (commercially available):

<u>Formula:</u>

Casein agar base

i-inositol . . . . 50.0 micrograms/ml
                                                                                      of medium

---

*The basal media and the media with added vitamins and amino acids are available from Difco Co., Detroit, Mich.

c. <u>Casein agar base plus thiamine-inositol</u> (commercially available):
   <u>Formula</u>:

   Casein agar base

   Thiamine hydrochloride. . . . . 0.2 micrograms/ml
   of medium

   i-inositol . . . . 50.0 micrograms/ml
   of medium

d. <u>Casein agar base plus thiamine</u> (commercially available):
   <u>Formula</u>:

   Casein agar base

   Thiamine hydrochloride. . . . . 0.2 micrograms/ml
   of medium

e. <u>Casein agar base plus nicotinic acid</u> (commercially available):
   <u>Formula</u>:

   Casein agar base

   Nicotinic acid . . . . 2.0 micrograms/ml
   of medium

f. <u>Ammonium nitrate agar base</u> (commercially available):
   <u>Formula</u>:

   Substitute 1.5 g of NH_4NO_3 for casein in the casein agar base medium.

g. <u>Ammonium nitrate agar base plus histidine</u> (commercially available):
   <u>Formula</u>:

   Ammonium nitrate agar base

   Histidine. . . . . 30.0 micrograms/ml
   of medium

   <u>Stock solutions*</u> - <u>vitamins</u>: After sterilizing for 10 minutes, store at 5° C.

   <u>Histidine solution</u> - 150.0 mg/100.0 ml distilled water

   <u>Inositol solution</u> - 250.0 mg/100.0 ml distilled water

   <u>Nicotinic acid solution</u> - 10.0 mg/100.0 ml distilled water

   <u>Thiamine solution</u> - 10.0 mg/1000 ml distilled water at a pH of 4-5

5. **Neutral Wort Agar** (commercially available): Medium for increasing spore production. Useful for production of macroconidia of *T. mentagrophytes* and *T. tonsurans*.
   <u>Formula</u>:

   Maltose. . . . . 12.75 g

   Malt extract . . . . 15.00 g

   Dextrin. . . . . 2.75 g

   Glycerol . . . . 2.35 g

   K_2HPO_4 . . . . 1.00 g

   NH_4Cl . . . . 1.00 g

   Peptone . . . . 0.78 g

*The use of 2 ml of the above stock solutions of vitamins will give the correct concentration for the preceding media for the differentiation of Trichophyton species.

Agar .... 15.00 g

Distilled water .... 1000.00 ml

Dissolve by heating to boiling, adjust pH to 6.8 or 7, tube, and autoclave for 10 minutes at 120° C.

6. **Rice Agar:** This preparation is used to differentiate *Microsporum audouinii* from *M. canis* and to stimulate conidial formation in some of the *Trichophyton* species.

Formula:

Unfortified rice .... 8 g

Water .... 25 ml

Autoclave at 15 lbs. for 15 minutes in an Erlenmeyer flask.

7. **Sabouraud Griseofulvin Medium** (Blank and Rebell, 1965): A medium for detecting griseofulvin-sensitive dermatophytes when compared with a standard Sabouraud glucose-chloramphenicol-cycloheximide medium.

Procedure:

To 1 liter of the hot commercial Sabouraud glucose-cycloheximide medium, add 20 mg of powdered griseofulvin, dissolved in 1 ml of acetone, tube, autoclave, and cool.

a. Use medium without griseofulvin for control tubes as organism will not grow in the medium containing griseofulvin if it is sensitive to the compound.

8. **Urease Test** (Philpot, 1967): This is a useful method for separation of *Trichophyton mentagrophytes* from *T. rubrum*. Within 7 days *T. mentagrophytes* strains should hydrolyze urea, and the medium becomes deep red, while *T. rubrum* is less rapid.

Formula (modification of Christensen's test medium):

Peptone .... 1 g

NaCl .... 5 g

KH_2PO_4 .... 2 g

Glucose .... 5 g

Agar .... 20 g

Distilled water .... 1000 ml

Dissolve by heat, add 5 ml of phenol red solution (0.2% in 50% alcohol). Autoclave at 115° C for 15 minutes, cool, and add 100 ml of urea (20% aqueous solution, sterilized by filtration). Tube and slant. Place a small amount of colony in the medium and incubate at 24°-26° C. Read in 7 days. A deep red color through the medium is a positive reaction.

G. Dimorphic Fungi: Media for development and maintenance of the dimorphic forms. In addition to brain-heart infusion agar and blood agar base media, other special media are useful:

1. **Cysteine Blood Agar:** Useful for development and maintenance of the yeast forms.

Formula:

10% rabbit or sheep blood agar with 1% dextrose and 0.1% cysteine.

2. **Salvin's YP Medium:** Especially useful for *Histoplasma capsulatum*.

Formula:

Proteose-peptone (Difco) .... 10.00 g

Neopeptone .... 3.25 g

Tryptone .... 3.25 g

Glucose	2.00 g
NaCl	5.00 g
Na_2HPO_4	2.50 g
Agar	1.75 g
Distilled water	1000.00 ml

Adjust pH to 6.5 to 7.5.

Dissolve by heat, tube, and sterilize.

3. **Sabhi Agar Base*** (Gorman, 1967): This medium with chloromycetin is useful for the recovery of *Blastomyces dermatitidis* and *Histoplasma capsulatum* from body tissues and fluids. The addition of 10% sheep or human blood increases the recovery of *H. capsulatum*. The cultures should be kept at room temperature (24° C) for up to 2 months. The Sabhi Agar Base with blood can be used to convert these two organisms to the yeast phase at 37° C.

Formula:

Calf brains, infusion from	100 g
Beef heart, infusion from	125 g
Bacto-proteose peptone	5 g
Bacto-neopeptone	5 g
Bacto-glucose	21 g
Sodium chloride	2.5 g
Disodium phosphate	1.25 g
Bacto-agar	15 g

To rehydrate the medium, suspend 59 g in 1000 ml of distilled water and heat to boiling. Sterilize in autoclave, cool to 50° C, and add 1 ml sterile 100 mg/ml chloromycetin solution. Dispense into tubes or plates.

Selected References

1. AJELLO, L., L. K. Georg, W. Kaplan and L. Kaufman. 1962. Laboratory Manual for Medical Mycology. PHSP. No. 994. Superintendent of Documents. U. S. Government Printing Office. Washington, D.C. 20402.
2. BARTELS, P. A., N. Wagoner and H. W. Larsh. 1968. Conversion of *Coccidioides immitis* in tissue culture. Mycopath. Mycol. app. 35:37
3. BAXTER, M. 1965. The use of blue ink in the identification of dermatophytes. J. Invest. Derm. 44:23.
4. BLANK, H. and G. Rebell. 1965. Griseofulvin medium for the diagnosis of dermatophytosis. Archs. Derm. 92(3):319.
5. BOJALIL, L. F. and J. Cerbon. 1959. Scheme for the differentiation of *Nocardia asteroides*, and *Nocardia brasiliensis*. J. Bact. 78:852.
6. BROSBE, E. A. 1967. Use of refined agar for the in vitro propagation of the spherule phase of *Coccidioides immitis*. J. Bact. 93:497.
7. CAMPBELL, C. C. 1945. Use of Francis' Glucose Cystine Blood Agar in the isolation and cultivation of *Sporotrichum schenckii*. J. Bact. 50:233.
8. COHEN, S. N. 1969. Modified Sabouraud medium containing neomycin and polymyxin. Appl. Microbiol. 17:486.

*Difco Laboratories, Detroit, Mich.

9. CONANT, N. F. 1936. Studies in the genus *Microsporum*. I. Cultural studies. Archs. Derm. 33:665.

10. CONANT, N. F. and R. A. Voge. 1954. The parasitic growth phase of *Coccidioides immitis* in culture. Mycologia 46:157.

11. EMMONS, C. W., C. H. Binford and J. P. Utz. 1963. Medical Mycology. Lea and Febiger. Philadelphia, Pa.

12. EVRON, R., and S. Ganor. 1968. The use of sodium taurocholate medium for identifying *Candida albicans*. J. Invest. Derm. 51:108.

13. FUENTES, C. A., F. Trespalacios, G. F. Baquero and R. Alboulafia. 1952. Effect of actidione on mold contaminants and on human pathogens. Mycologia 44:170.

14. GEORG, L. K., L. Ajello and C. Papageorge. 1954. Use of cycloheximide in the selective isolation of fungi pathogenic to man. J. Lab. Clin. Med. 44:422.

15. GEORG, L. K. and L. B. Camp. 1957. Routine nutritional test for the identification for dermatophytes. J. Bact. 74:113.

16. GORMAN, J. W. 1967. Sabhi, a new culture medium for pathogenic fungi. Am. J. Med. Tech. 33:151.

17. HALEY, L. D. 1964. Diagnostic Medical Mycology. Appleton-Century-Crofts. New York, N. Y.

18. HAZEN, E. L. 1947. The effect of yeast extract, thiamine, pyridoxine and *Bacillus weidmaniensis* on the colony characteristics and macroconidial formation. Mycologia. 39:200.

19. LEWIS, G. M., W. Sachs and M. E. Hopper. 1951. Mycologic and histologic techniques in the study of superficial fungous infections. Arch. Dermat. and Syph. 63:622.

20. LITTMAN, M. L. 1955. Liver-spleen glucose blood agar for *Histoplasma capsulatum* and other fungi. Am. J. Clin. Path. 25:1148.

21. Mc CLUNG, N. M. 1960. Isolation of *Nocardia asteroides* from soils. Mycologia 52:154.

22. Mc DONOUGH, E. S., L. Ajello, L. K. Georg and S. Brinkman. 1960. *In vitro* effects of antibiotics on yeast phase of *Blastomyces dermatitidis* and other fungi. J. Lab. Clin. Med. 55:116.

23. Mc DONOUGH, E. S., L. K. Georg, L. Ajello and S. Brinkman. 1960. Growth of dimorphic human pathogenic fungi on media containing cycloheximide and chloramphenicol. Mycopathologia. 13:113.

24. MISHRA, S. K. and H. S. Randhawa. 1969. Application of paraffin bait technique to the isolation of *Nocardia asteroides* from clinical specimens. Appl. Microbiol. 18:686.

25. PHILPOT, C. 1967. The differentiation of *Trichophyton mentagrophytes* from *T. rubrum* by a simple urease test. Sabouraudia 5:189.

26. SALVIN, S. B. 1947. Cultural studies on the yeastlike phase of *Histoplasma capsulatum* Darling. J. Bact. 54:655.

27. SEELIGER, H. 1955. Ein neues Medium zur Pseudomycelbildung von *Candida albicans*. Zeitscher. F. Hygiene 141:488.

28. SMITH, C. E., E. G. Whiting, E. E. Baker, H. G. Rosenberger, R. R. Beard and M. T. Saito. 1948. The use of coccidioidin. Am. Rev. Tuberc. 57:330.

29. TASCHDJIAN, C. L. 1957. Routine identification of *Candida albicans:* Current methods and a new medium. Mycologia 59:332.

30. TASCHDJIAN, C. L., J. J. Burchall and P. J. Kozinn. 1960. Rapid identification of *Candida albicans* by filamentation of serum and serum substitutes. J. Dis. Child. 99:212.

31. TAPLIN, D., N. Zaias, G. Rebell and H. Blank. 1969. Isolation and recognition of dermatophytes on a new medium (DTM). Archs. Derm. 99:203.

32. VOGEL, R. A. 1969. Primary isolation medium for *Cryptococcus neoformans*. Appl. Microbiol. 18:1100.

33. WEITZMAN, I. and M. Silva-Hutner. 1967. Nonkeratinous agar media as substrates for the ascigerous state in certain members of the Gymnoascaceae pathogenic for man and animals. Sabouraudia 5:335.

34. WIEGAND, S. E., J. A. Ulrich and R. K. Winkelmann. 1968. Diagnosis of superficial pathogenic fungi; use of ink blue method. Mayo Clin. Proc. 43:795.

Animal Inoculations

The inoculation of the laboratory animal is of value in establishing the pathogenicity of fungi, as well as for observation of the tissue phase characteristics of some of the pathogenic fungi. In some cases where infected material failed to grow in culture, the material may develop disease symptoms in the animals. Information on inoculation of animals with a specific pathogenic fungus is listed under procedures for that organism in the manual.

Types of Animals Used

Some of the more commonly used laboratory animals are mice, guinea pigs, rabbits, and hamsters.

Method of Inoculation

Animals are inoculated either intracerebrally, intravenously, intraperitoneally, or intratesticularly with saline suspensions of the organism using a syringe and the proper size needle. Equipment should be sterilized prior to use and care should be taken to see that all of the suspension is put into the animal. Disinfect equipment used during the inoculation of the animals. For mice the following quantities of the saline suspension may be sufficient for injection, depending upon concentrations:

1. **Intracerebral:** About 0.25 ml suspension of the organisms in a tuberculin syringe with a 26-gauge needle. The needle is inserted posteriorly to the right of the midline of the skull, penetrating only slightly inside.

2. **Intravenous:** 0.2 ml or less depending on concentration with a 1 ml or smaller syringe and a 26-gauge needle. The inoculum should be injected into one of the four veins in the mouse's tail.

3. **Intraperitoneal:** About 0.5 ml suspension of the organisms in a 1 ml or larger syringe and a 24-gauge needle. The needle is inserted through the skin and peritoneum, but not deep into the abdominal cavity.

Animals should be sacrificed periodically to observe the course of the infection.

Gastric Mucin

A 5% hog gastric mucin may enhance the virulence of the fungi when the suspension is inoculated into the animal.

Procedure:

1. Put 5 g of gastric mucin in 95 ml of distilled water; emulsify with a Waring Blender for 5 minutes.

2. Autoclave for 15 minutes at 120° C; cool.

3. Adjust pH to 7.3 with NaOH (sterile).

4. Check for sterility and store in refrigerator.

5. Use equal parts of the gastric mucin and the fungus suspension and inject the mixture (1 ml) intraperitoneally into the laboratory animal.

Isolation of Pathogenic Fungi from Soil Utilizing Mice

Soil screening through laboratory animals, especially mice, has been one of the most fruitful methods for increasing knowledge concerning the natural habitats of pathogenic fungi. A number of modified procedures have been used including variations in the ratio of the soil sample to the physiological saline solution, variations in the antibiotics used, and in the length of time to hold the mice prior to sacrifice and culture of fungi from internal organs.

<u>Procedure for Isolation</u> (References: Ajello, 1960; Emmons, 1961).

1. A sample of soil is taken by pressing the open mouth of a sterile 4 oz screw-cap bottle or large test tube against the surface of the superficial layer of soil and scooping up the sample.

2. Make up a soil and physiological solution in the proportion of about 1:5, without antibiotics.

3. After thoroughly stirring or shaking the suspension of soil, the sample is allowed to settle for about 1 hour.

4. An 8-ml portion of the supernatant is removed and combined with 2 ml of an antibiotic solution (2 mg streptomycin and 5 mg penicillin per ml of water).

5. One-ml suspensions are injected intraperitoneally into a total of 5 mice.

6. Sacrifice the mice in 1 month.

7. Isolate portions of infected spleen, omentum, liver, or other organs on modified Sabouraud agar with antibiotics, or other media. Mince the tissue with scissors, spread with inoculating needle, and incubate at 24° C for 4 weeks.

Embryonated Hen's Egg

This medium has been found useful in the primary isolation and tissue phase culture of some of the fungi. The yolk sac is recommended as the site of inoculation.

Selected References

1. AJELLO, L. 1960. *Histoplasma capsulatum* soil studies. Mykosen 3:43.
2. BRUECK, J. W. and F. J. Buddingh. 1951. Propagation of pathogenic fungi in the yolk sac of embryonated eggs. Proc. Soc. Exper. Biol. and Med. 76:258.
3. EMMONS, C. W. 1961. Isolation of *Histoplasma capsulatum* from soil in Washington, D. C. Public Health Reports 76:591.
4. HALEY, L. D. 1964. Diagnostic Medical Mycology. Chapter 20. Appleton-Century-Crofts. New York.
5. STRAUSS, R. E. and A. M. Kligman. 1951. The use of gastric mucin to lower resistance of laboratory animals to systemic fungus infections. J. Infect. Dis. 88:151.
6. VOGEL, R. A. and N. F. Conant. 1952. The cultivation of *Coccidioides immitis* in the embryonated hen's egg. J. Bact. 64:83.

Maintenance of Stock Cultures of Fungi

There are several ways to maintain culture collections. With the exception of lyophilization, all methods are easy to do without special equipment.

1. **Room Temperature** (22-24° C): Stock cultures are maintained in racks or baskets for up to 3 months before subculturing. The length of time before the media dry out and consequent

death of the cultures, varies, depending upon the type of plug, relative humidity, and the size of the test tube. A sealed or capped tube will not dry out as rapidly.

2. **Refrigeration** (5-10° C): Stock cultures may be maintained for up to 4 months before transferring to new slants as the tubes dry out more slowly. Capped tubes or sealed tubes usually may be kept for 6 months. Some of the *Trichophyton* species that do not produce microconidia readily, *Epidermophyton floccosum,* and *Microsporum audouinii* should be maintained at room temperature, as they usually die when refrigerated.

3. **Deep Freeze** (-20° C or lower): This method is satisfactory for most fungi that sporulate. After growth of the fungus on phytone yeast extract agar recommended by Carmichael (1962) or on other media such as Mycophil agar for 10 to 14 days, the tubes with caps tightened are placed in the freezer at approximately -20° C. Viability should be maintained for a number of years by this method.

4. **Mineral Oil**: The stock culture is maintained by pouring sterile mineral oil (Saybolt viscosity 330 at 100° F) over the entire agar slant containing an actively growing colony. The entire agar surface must be completely covered to prevent loss of water from the medium. The cultures may be viable for several years when kept in an upright position.

   To make a transfer, a small portion of the fungus is removed from below the surface of the mineral oil and, after excess oil drains off, is placed in a new agar slant.

   About 100 ml of mineral oil in a flask should be sterilized for 45 minutes at 120° C before use.

5. **Lyophilization**: This method is excellent for certain types of fungi to preserve them in a stable condition for an indefinite number of years. Many small spored fungi such as *Penicillium* sp., *Aspergillus* sp., some of the yeasts, *Actinomyces* sp., and other microorganisms have been preserved for years by this method. A number of the large spored or poorly sporulating pathogenic fungi are not very suitable for lyophilization. The procedure may be found under Selected References (Hesseltine, 1960; Fennell, 1960; Raper and Alexander, 1945; Tuite, 1969).

6. **Cryogenic Storage**: This method is increasing in usage as small liquid nitrogen refrigerators are presently available for a reasonable price (Linde Division, Union Carbide, Tonawanda, N.Y., and Cryogenic Engineering Co., Denver, Colo.). This method is particularly useful for organisms that do not survive well when lyophilized. More information may be found under Selected References (Tuite, 1968, 1969; Hwang, 1966; Muggelton, 1964).

Selected References

1. CARMICHAEL, J. W. 1962. Viability of mold cultures stored at -20° C. Mycologia 54:432.
2. FENNELL, Dorothy, 1960. Conservation of fungous cultures. Bot. Rev. 26:79.
3. HESSELTINE, C. W., B. J. Bradle and C. R. Benjamin. 1960. Further investigations on the preservation of molds. Mycologia 52:762.
4. HWANG, S. W. 1966. Effects of ultra-low temperatures on the viability of selected fungus strains. Mycologia 52:527.
5. MUGGLETON, P. W. 1964. The preservation of cultures. Prog. Ind. Microbiol. 4:190.
6. RAPER, K. B. and D. F. Alexander. 1945. Preservation of molds by the lyophil process. Mycologia 37:499.
7. TESH, R. B., J. D. Schneidau and C. A. Erwin. 1967. The effect of freezing and storage at -24° C on the survival of pathogenic fungi in excised tissue. Am. J. Clin. Path. 48:100.
8. TUITE, J. 1969. Plant Pathological Methods. Fungi and Bacteria. Burgess Publishing Co., Minneapolis, Minn.
9. WERHANM, C. C. 1946. Mineral oil as a fungus culture preservative. Mycologia 38:691.

SUPERFICIAL MYCOSES
EXTERNAL OTITIS

(Otomycosis, Myringomycosis, Fungus Ear, Hot Weather Ear)

Definition:

External otitis is a mild or chronic infection of the external ear characterized by itching, inflammation, and an accumulation of large masses of epithelial debris containing either bacteria or fungi, or both. A minority of cases are caused by fungi, while the majority of cases are caused by bacteria.

Etiological Agents:

A total of 53 species of fungi have been reported as agents of external otitis. Probably less than 10% of the cases are caused by fungi as the primary invaders. Some of the more frequently reported genera are: *Aspergillus, Penicillium, Mucor,* and *Rhizopus.* Bacteria most frequently isolated as the primary cause are: *Pseudomonas, Micrococcus, Staphylococcus, Streptococcus, Proteus,* and others.

Occurrence:

1. **Man:** The disease is worldwide in distribution, especially in the tropical and subtropical regions, and is more prevalent in the southern and southwestern parts of the United States.

2. **Animals:** External otitis does occur and probably is due to many of the same organisms as in man.

Laboratory Procedures

1. **Source of Infected Material:** Using sterile techniques to avoid contamination, and under the supervision of a physician, especially in the case of deep-seated infections, the exudate and debris should be removed and streaked on culture media as soon as possible, or placed in a sterile vial for examination as soon as facilities are available.

2. **Examination of Infected Material:**

   a. Place the epithelial debris on a slide in a drop of 10% potassium hydroxide (KOH), and examine after adding a cover glass. The exudate should be stained by Gram method (see staining procedures, page 32) and examined for the presence of bacteria.

   b. Microscopically, fungi should appear in the KOH preparation as fragments of mycelium, with or without branches and septa, and in some cases conidiophores and spores may be present. Direct demonstration is more diagnostic than cultures as contaminants may be present.

   Microscopically, bacteria that are present on the stained slide may be *Pseudomonas* or *Proteus* if gram negative rods, or *Streptococcus* or *Micrococcus* if gram positive. Coliform bacilli, diphtheroids and others may be present on the stained slide. Cultures should be made for identification of the organisms.

3. **Cultures:**

   a. For fungi, the material from the ear should be streaked on Sabouraud glucose agar plates or slants and held for 2 to 3 weeks, as most saprophytic fungi develop during this time.

      (1) A portion of the colony should be removed and placed on a slide with lactophenol; if too thick, tease apart and put on a cover glass. The cellophane tape-cover glass mount

will keep more of the reproductive structures of the fungus intact for identification. Look for conidiophores (or sporangiophores) and conidia (or spores), septate or non-septate hyphae, or any other clues for identification of the saprophytic fungus. Check the section on contaminants, or reference books that contain thousands of the Fungi Imperfecti for identifications. In many cases isolates will be species of *Aspergillus, Penicillium, Mucor* or *Rhizopus.* In some cases pathogenic fungi causing dermatomycosis have been isolated.

b. <u>For bacteria</u>, suitable media, such as nutrient agar, tryptose soybean broth, blood agar, etc., should be streaked and incubated at 37° C. The predominant organism or organisms should be identified. If *Micrococcus* is the predominant organism, a coagulase test should be run, and if the results are positive, the organism is considered pathogenic. Sensitivity tests to penicillin, streptomycin, terramycin, chloromycetin, erythromycin, sulfanilamide, sulfadiazine, and other antibiotics that are available should be run to determine the proper choice for treatment, as many organisms have become resistant to these therapeutic agents. More frequently isolated bacteria are: *Pseudomonas, Streptococcus, Micrococcus,* and *Proteus.*

4. **Animal Inoculation:** Not necessary for establishing pathogenicity.

<u>Questions:</u>

1. Why is otomycosis an inaccurate description for this disease?

2. Of what value are bacterial sensitivity tests to the physician?

Selected References

1. FORKNER, C. E., Jr. 1960. *Pseudomonas aeruginosa* infections. Grune & Stratton. New York. Pp. 60-63.
2. HALEY, L. D. 1952. Etiology of otomycosis. I. Mycologic flora of the ear. II. Bacterial flora of the ear. III. Observations on attempts to induce otomycosis in rabbits. IV. Clinical observations. Arch. Otolaryng. 52:202, 208, 214, 220.
3. JONES, E. H. and P. G. McLain. 1962. Fungal infections of external ear canal. Southern Med. J. 55:910.
4. JONES, E. H. 1965. External Otitis: Diagnosis and Treatment. Charles C. Thomas, Publisher. Springfield, Ill.
5. McGONIGLE, J. J. and O. F. Jillson. 1967. Otomycosis: an entity. Archs. Derm. 95:45.
6. RUSH-MUNRO, F. M. 1966. *Allescheria boydii (Monosporium apiospermum)* associated with cases of otomycosis in New Zealand. N. Z. J. Med. Lab. Tech. 20:3.
7. SINGER, D. E., E. Freeman, W. R. Hoffert, R. V. Keys, R. B. Mitchell and A. V. Hardy. 1952. Otitis externa. Bacteriological and mycological studies. Ann. Otol. Rhin. and Laryng. 61:317.
8. STUART, E. A. and F. Blank. 1955. Aspergillosis of the ear. A report of twenty-nine cases. Canad. Med. Assoc. J. 72:334.
9. WOLF, F. T. 1947. Relation of various fungi to otomycosis. Arch. Otolaryng. 46:361.

PIEDRA

(Black Piedra, White Piedra, Tinea Nodosa)

Definition:

Piedra is a fungus infection on the hair in the form of small stony nodules. Black piedra affects the hair of the scalp, while white piedra involves the hairs of the beard and mustache. White piedra has lighter brown-colored nodules that are less firmly attached to the hair shaft.

Etiological Agents:

Piedraia hortai (Brumpt) Fonseca and Arêa Leão; 1928, causes black piedra; *Trichosporon beigelii* (Rabenhorst) Vuillemin, 1902, causes white piedra.

Occurrence:

1. **Man:** Black piedra is found chiefly in South America, Southern Asia, and Indonesia. White piedra is reported in South America, Central Europe, Japan, England, the Orient, and, in a few cases, the United States.

2. **Animals:** Black piedra was reported in monkeys and a chimpanzee. White piedra has been reported in horses, chimpanzee pelts, and in a black spider monkey.

Laboratory Procedures

1. **Source of Infected Material:** If cases are available, the hairs with the stony nodules should be cut off and placed in a sterile container or an envelope for examination.

2. **Examination of Infected Material:**

   a. Place infected hair on a slide containing a drop of 10% potassium hydroxide (KOH) or lactophenol and add a cover glass. Slides with lactophenol may be sealed with fingernail polish.

   b. Microscopically, the nodules caused by *P. hortai* vary in size and shape. This somatic structure is a tightly formed stroma of dark brown, dichotomously branched hyphae, 4-8 μ in diameter. Numerous septations in the hyphae with thick walls gives the appearance of arthrospores. (See Plate I.) If the nodule is broken apart, numerous asci may be seen with 2 to 8 ascospores that are fusiform, slightly curved, with a polar filament at each end, or sometimes the spores are considered to be banana-shaped.

   Microscopically, the nodules caused by *T. beigelii* vary in size and are softer and more easily separated from the hair shaft than *P. hortai* (see Plate I). This somatic structure is a transparent, greenish-brown mycelial mass which forms round to rectangular cells, usually 2-4 μ in diameter, in the hyphal strands. Hyphae separate into oval arthrospores, but no asci are formed.

3. **Cultures:**

   P. hortai: Colonies develop readily from hairs placed on Sabouraud glucose agar with cycloheximide at room temperature.

   a. *P. hortai* in culture develops a greenish-brown to black colony which is raised in the center or is flat, and glabrous to cerebriform (see Plate I).

      (1) Microscopically, the hyphae are dark, thick-walled, closely septate, with numerous chlamydospores or enlarged irregular cells. Asci and ascospores may form in culture.

   T. beigelii: Colonies grow rapidly from hairs placed on Sabouraud glucose agar. The organism is sensitive to cycloheximide.

54

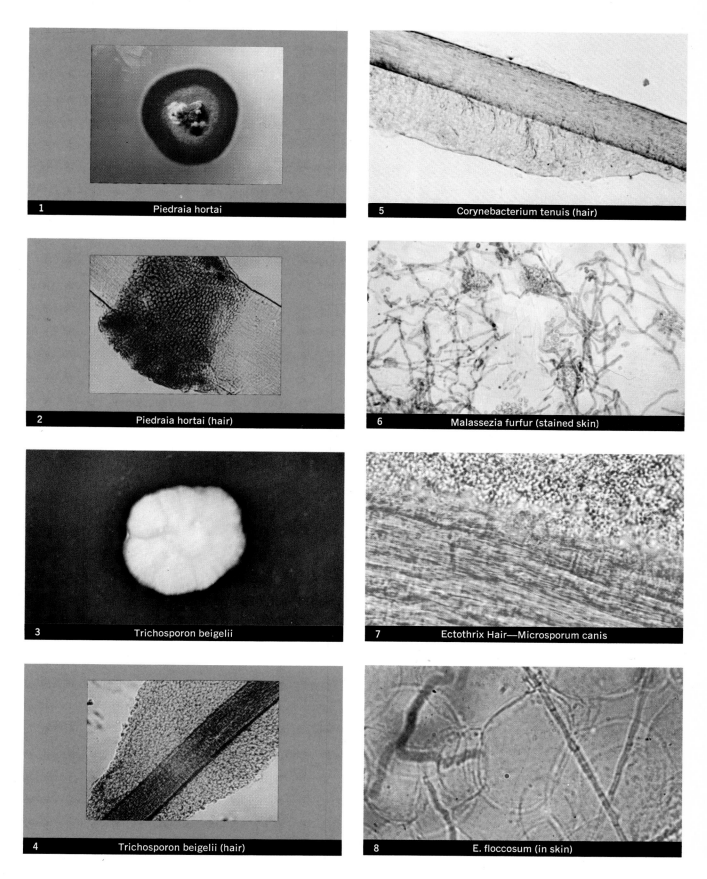

1   Piedraia hortai

5   Corynebacterium tenuis (hair)

2   Piedraia hortai (hair)

6   Malassezia furfur (stained skin)

3   Trichosporon beigelii

7   Ectothrix Hair—Microsporum canis

4   Trichosporon beigelii (hair)

8   E. floccosum (in skin)

PLATE I

Biochemical tests necessary for species determination: *T. beigelii* will not ferment sugars; it will assimilate glucose, galactose, sucrose, lactose, and maltose. Arbutin is split, but potassium nitrate is not assimilated.

a. *T. beigelii* in culture develops rapidly as a cream-colored, slimy, soft colony, later becoming finely wrinkled, raised in the center, darker, and more firmly attached to the agar (see Plate I).

   (1) <u>Microscopically</u>, the hyphae may contain blastospores when colonies are young, later the hyphae form many arthrospores. No asci are formed.

4. **Animal Inoculation:** Laboratory animals are not successfully infected.

<u>Questions</u>:

1. How can black and white piedra be differentiated from trichomycosis axillaris on the hair shaft?

2. Compare with an ectothrix or mosaic hair infection.

Selected References

1. AREA LEÃO, A. E. 1941. Considerações sôbre os thallosporados. O gênero *Trichosporon*. Mem. Inst. Oswaldo Cruz. 35:729.
2. DALY, J. F. 1957. Piedra in Vermont. A. M. A. Arch. Dermat. 75:584.
3. HORTA, P. 1911. Sôbre una nova forma de piedra. Mem. Inst. Oswaldo Cruz. 3:87.
4. KAPLAN, W. 1959. Piedra in lower animals. J. Am. Vet. Med. Assoc. 134:113.
5. LONDERO, A. T., C. D. Ramos and O. Fischman. 1966. White piedra of unusual localization. Sabouraudia 5:132.
6. LOCHTE, T. 1937. Über das vorkommen der piedra beim schimpansen und über die beziehungen der tierischen piedra zur menschlichen. Arch. Derm. u. Syph. 175:107.
7. PATTERSON, J. C., S. L. Laine and W. B. Taylor. 1962. White piedra. Arch. Dermat. 85:534.

TINEA VERSICOLOR

(Pityriasis Versicolor, Liver Spots)

Definition:

Tinea versicolor is a superficial infection of the horny layer of the epidermis characterized by irregular fawn to brown, or at times achromatic, scaly patches principally on the chest or back, and occasionally on arms, thighs, groin, neck, axillae, or face (Plate III, Figs. 73 & 74).

Etiological Agent:

Malassezia furfur (Robin) Baillon, 1889. *Pityrosporum ovale* and *P. orbiculare* are probably synonymous.

Occurrence:

1. **Man:** The disease comprises not over 5% of the fungus diseases in temperate regions, but is much more frequent in the tropical areas throughout the world. Cases have occurred after large doses of ACTH or corticosteroids.

2. **Animals:** No record of an infection.

Laboratory Procedures

1. **Source of Infected Material:** The fawn to brown patches should be scraped with a scalpel and collected on a slide or in a container for examination. Cellulose tapes may be pressed against the skin to obtain the scales for examination.

2. **Examination of Infected Material:**

   a. To locate all areas of infection on the skin, Wood's light may be used. Infected lesions show a pale yellow fluorescence under dark conditions. Furfuraceous scales will show some fluorescence after removal from the lesions.

   b. Place scales in a drop of 10% potassium hydroxide on a slide and add a cover glass. Heat gently and examine. A little blue-black ink may be added to color the somatic structures of the fungus (see procedures, page 29).

      (1) Other procedures: Thin scales may be mounted in a drop of lactophenol with cotton blue, a drop of methylene blue, or fixed to a slide and stained with the periodic acid-Schiff method (Kligman's modification, see procedures page 30). Other stains, including Gram and acridine orange stains, may be used.

   c. Procedure for direct staining on vinyl plastic tape (Keddie, Orr and Liebes, 1961):

      (1) Pieces of Scotch brand tapes containing infected fragments of the horny layer of the skin, can be held with a forceps and transferred through the solutions for staining. After staining, the adhesive side is mounted toward the cover glass. (The adhesive side of the tape may be put up on a slide and drops of the stain may be used in place of submerging the piece of tape into solutions.)

   d. Acridine Orange Stain (Bertalanffy, 1960):

      Procedure:

      (1) Fix in 100% alcohol 1 minute, dip in 1% acetic acid, and finally in distilled H_2O.

      (2) Stain in acridine orange solution - 3 minutes.

      (3) Remove excess stain in phosphate buffer - 1-2 minutes.

(4) Differentiate in 1/10 molar calcium chloride - 1-2 minutes.

(5) Dehydrate, clear, and mount in Harleco synthetic resin, balsam, or a nonfluorescent synthetic mounting medium.

(6) Check the fluorescent fungus elements and epithelial cells (green and orange) under a fluorescent microscope.

Stock Stain:

Acridine orange (C. I. 46005, National Aniline Div., Allied Chemical Corporation, New York).

0.1% aqueous acridine orange solution diluted to 0.01% with phosphate buffer pH 6.0.

e. Microscopically, the organisms appear as clusters of thick-walled, round cells, 3 to 8 μ in diameter. Some may be budding forms. Numerous short, straight, or angular hyphae may surround the clusters (Plate I, Fig. 6).

3. **Cultures:**

a. Routinely, cultures are not necessary. Cultures obtained by Gordon (1951) on Sabouraud glucose agar with olive oil on the surface are *Pityrosporum orbiculare*. *Malassezia furfur* and *P. orbiculare* are similar but have not been shown to be identical (Sternberg and Keddie, 1961; and Keddie et al, 1963).

4. **Animal Inoculation:** Laboratory animals are not successfully infected.

5. **Histopathology:**

a. The organism will grow abundantly in the deeper layers of the stratum corneum. Histological sections readily show the organism after being stained with hematoxylin and eosin, Giemsa, methylene blue, or periodic acid-Schiff stain.

Question:

1. How does tinea nigra differ from tinea versicolor?

Selected References

1. BURKE, R. C. 1961. Tinea versicolor: Susceptibility factors and experimental infection in human beings. J. Invest. Dermat. 36:389.
2. COHEN, M. M. 1954. A simple procedure for staining tinea versicolor (*M. furfur*) with fountain pen ink. J. Invest. Dermat. 22:9.
3. GORDON, M. A. 1951. Lipophilic yeastlike organisms associated with tinea versicolor. J. Invest. Dermat. 17:267.
4. HANTSCHKE, D. and K. Nischio. 1968. Laborinfektion durch *Malassezia furfur*. Mykosen 11:235.
5. KEDDIE, R., A. Orr and D. Liebes. 1961. Direct staining on vinyl plastic tape, demonstrating the cutaneous flora of the epidermis by the strip method. Sabouraudia 1:108.
6. KEDDIE, F. and S. Shadomy. 1963. Etiological significance of *Pityrosporum orbiculare* in tinea versicolor. Sabouraudia 3:21.
7. STERNBERG, T. H. and F. Keddie. 1961. Immunofluorescence studies in tinea versicolor. Archs. Derm. 84:999.

TRICHOMYCOSIS AXILLARIS

(Leptothrix, Trichomycosis Nodosa)

Definition:

Trichomycosis axillaris is an infection of the axillary and pubic hairs. Yellow, red, or black concretions develop around the hair shaft (Plate I, Fig. 5).

Etiological Agent:

Corynebacterium tenuis (Castellani) Crissey *et al*, 1952 (*Nocardia tenuis* Castellani, 1912) or two or three species of diphtheroids.

Occurrence:

1. **Man:** Common in temperate climate, more widespread in the tropics.
2. **Animals:** No record of an infection.

Laboratory Procedures

1. **Source of Infected Material:** Collect axillary or pubic hairs with nodules scattered along the hair shaft. Note color and lack of luster.

2. **Examination of Infected Material:**

   a. Place infected hairs under Wood's ultraviolet light and note pale yellow color when concretion is yellow.

   b. Place infected hairs on a slide containing a drop of 10% potassium hydroxide (KOH) or lactophenol and add a cover glass. Heat gently to clear more rapidly. Slides with lactophenol may be sealed with fingernail polish.

   c. Microscopically, the concretions sometimes show short bacillary forms not over 1μ in diameter (Plate I, Fig. 5) or black forms have clumps of cocci mixed with bacillary forms (usually *Micrococcus castellani* and *M. nigrescens*). Crushed material may be Gram-stained.

3. **Cultures:** Culture is not necessary for diagnosis. After immersion of hair with granules in 70% alcohol for 1 second, the granules are soaked in buffered saline overnight and cultured. Casman's sheep blood agar (Difco) or brain-heart infusion agar with 1% Tween 80 may be used. Incubate for 7 days at 37° C. Cultures of diphtheroids should develop.

4. **Animal Inoculation:** Laboratory animals are not susceptible.

Questions:

1. Compare the microscopic appearance of trichomycosis axillaris with white and black piedra. Any differences? Compare with infected hairs from tinea capitis cases.

Selected References

1. CRISSEY, J. T., G. C. Rebell and J. J. Laskas. 1952. Studies on the causative organism of trichomycosis axillaris. J. Invest. Dermat. 19:187.
2. FREEMAN, R. G., M. E. McBride and J. M Knox. 1969. Pathogenesis of trichomycosis axillaris. Archs. Derm. 100:90.
3. McBRIDE, M. E., R. G. Freeman and J. M. Knox. 1968. A method for the isolation of the causative organisms of trichomycosis axillaris. Brit. J. Derm. 80:509.

TINEA NIGRA

(Pityriasis Nigra, Microsporosis Nigra)

Definition:

Tinea nigra is a superficial fungus infection of the palm of the hands, rarely found on the neck or other parts of the body. It is characterized by brown to black macular lesions on the skin (Plate III, Figs. 71 & 72).

Etiological Agent:

Cladosporium werneckii Horta, 1921. Probably occurs in the soil and on wood or paint in warm climates. There is a close resemblance to *Aureobasidium (Pullularia) pullulans* in the early stages of colony formation. Infection probably occurs from injection of the skin with contaminated materials.

Occurrence:

1. **Man:** The disease has been reported from Central America, South America, Southeast Asia, Indonesia, and United States.

2. **Animals:** No record of infection.

Laboratory Procedures

1. **Source of Infected Material:** Scrapings should be taken from pigmented lesions of tinea nigra for examination microscopically and for culture, or placed in a sterile container for laboratory study.

2. **Examination of Infected Material:**

   a. Place scrapings on a slide with 10% KOH and examine microscopically.

   b. <u>Microscopically</u>, the fungus appears in the epithelial cells of the skin as pigmented, light brown to dark green, branched, septate hyphae between 1.5 to 3μ in diameter. Swollen cells and chlamydospores should be seen.

3. **Cultures:**

   a. Infected material will grow on Sabouraud glucose agar with or without the addition of cycloheximide and chloramphenicol at room temperature. A 3-week period should be allowed for growth before being considered negative.

   b. Colonies develop slowly with a moist, shiny black, yeastlike appearance, reaching maximum size after two weeks. These older colonies have less moisture on the surface, and become dark green with grayish mycelium on the surface. Transfers develop the yeastlike growth at first, but soon become blackish with aerial mycelium.

   c. Microscopically, the black yeastlike portion of the colony contains blastospores or budding cells which have developed laterally from the dark hyphal cells.

   Blastospores may form clusters along the hyphae (similar to *Aureobasidium* sp. and *Candida* sp.). Short conidiophores on the sides or apices of the hyphae produce chains or clusters of 1- to 2-celled dark conidia. This simulates spore formation in *Cladosporium* (or *Hormodendrum*). Older hyphae may lack spores, or have conidiophores of the Cladosporium type.

4. **Animal Inoculation:** Animal infection is of no value in laboratory diagnosis of the disease. Superficial infection can be produced experimentally in guinea pigs, or by intraperitoneal injection of the organism in mice, and recovered a few days later.

<u>Questions:</u>

1. What are the differences and similarities in the hyphae and conidia of the genera *Aureobasidium, Candida* and *Cladosporium (Hormodendrum)?*

2. Compare the appearance of the hyphae in skin scrapings from tinea nigra and tinea corporis cases. Are there any microscopic differences?

Selected References

1. CASTELLANI, A. and A. J. Chalmers. 1919. Manual of Tropical Medicine. 3rd Edition. Bailliere, Tindall and Cox, London.
2. COOKE, W. B. 1959. An ecological life history of *Aureobasidium pullulans* (de Bary) Arnaud. Mycopathologia. 12:1.
3. GOMEZ, S. H., J. V. Cardenas and P. I. Rendon. 1968. Tinea nigra. Mycopath. Mycol. appl. 34:11.
4. KEDDIE, F. 1964. *Cladosporium wernickii:* infection and in vivo culture. Archs. Derm. 89: 432.
5. MERWIN, C. F. 1965. Tinea nigra palmaris. Review of literature and case report. Pediatrics, Springfield 36:537.
6. RITCHIE, E. B. and T. E. Taylor. 1964. A study of tinea nigra palmaris. Archs. Derm. 89: 601.
7. VAN VELSOR, H. and H. Singetary. 1964. Tinea nigra palmaris, a report of 15 cases from coastal North Carolina. Archs. Derm. 90(1):59.
8. WALSH, E. N. 1948. Tinea nigra in Panama. Archs. Derm. and Syph. 57:732.

DERMATOMYCOSES

Introduction

The dermatomycoses are a group of fungus infections of the skin caused by a definite group of fungi known as dermatophytes. These organisms invade the keratinized areas of the body such as the skin, hair, and nails, and are the most common and widely distributed of the fungus diseases. They are rarely found in the subcutaneous tissues or internal organs of the body. The diseases they produce are known as ringworms or tineas. These diseases are incited by species of three genera: *Microsporum, Epidermophyton,* and *Trichophyton.* Cutaneous moniliasis which may resemble the tineas is usually caused by *Candida* sp. The isolation and identification of the species of the fungus from skin or nail scrapings or from stubs of infected hairs are essential where cases have been difficult to treat medically.

Classification

The classification of the dermatomycoses is based on two systems. The clinical symptomatology involving various areas of the body is one classification system. This is used before identification of the fungus can be determined as the same species can produce similar symptoms in different parts of the body. The other system is based on morphological characteristics of the fungus with separation of genera based on the shape of the macroconidia (fuseaux).

DISEASE	FUNGUS
Tinea capitis (Ringworm of scalp) (Plate II, Figs. 51-60)	*Microsporum* - any species *Trichophyton* - any species except 　　*T. concentricum*
Tinea barbae (Ringworm of the beard, 　　Barber's itch) (Plate III, Fig. 70)	*Trichophyton mentagrophytes* *Trichophyton rubrum* *Trichophyton violaceum* *Trichophyton verrucosum* *Microsporum canis*
Tinea corporis (Ringworm of the body) (Plate II & III, Figs. 61-69)	*Trichophyton mentagrophytes* *Trichophyton rubrum* *Trichophyton concentricum* 　　(Tinea imbricata) *Microsporum audouinii* *Microsporum canis* Any of the other dermatophytes may be 　　involved
Tinea cruris (Jockey itch, gym itch, 　　ringworm of the groin) (Plate III, Figs. 78, 79, & 87)	*Epidermophyton floccosum* *Trichophyton mentagrophytes* *Trichophyton rubrum* 　　(*Candida albicans*)
Tinea pedis (Athlete's foot, 　　ringworm of the feet) (Plate III, Figs. 77, 81, 82, 84 & 85)	*Epidermophyton floccosum* *Trichophyton mentagrophytes* *Trichophyton rubrum* 　　(*Candida albicans*)

<u>DISEASE</u>	<u>FUNGUS</u>
Tinea unguium (Onychomycosis, ringworm of the nail) (Plate III, Figs. 81 & 90)	*Trichophyton mentagrophytes* *Trichophyton rubrum* Rare: *T. violaceum, T. schoenleinii, T. tonsurans*
Ringworm in Animals: (attacks skin, hair, feathers, nails, claws and hooves) (Fig. 40)	*Microsporum canis* *Microsporum gypseum* *Trichophyton mentagrophytes* *Trichophyton verrucosum*
Favus in Animals (Tinea favosa)	*Trichophyton equinum* *Trichophyton gallinae* Rare: *M. audouinii, M. distortum, M. cookei, M. nanum, M. van-breuseghemii, T. ajelloi, T. rubrum, T. schoenleinii*

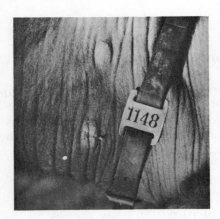

Figure 40. Tinea on cow

Mycological Classification of the Dermatophytes

This group of fungi originally was represented by three genera: *Microsporum, Epidermophyton,* and *Trichophyton* which were separated by Emmons in 1934 on the basis of differences in the macroconidia. Recently Ajello (1968) transferred the species in the genus *Keratinomyces* to *Trichophyton* on the basis of microconidia and the perfect state.

Most of the dermatophytes have been considered Deuteromycetes (Fungi Imperfecti) until the discovery of the ascigerous state in *K. ajelloi* (Dawson and Gentles, 1961) and *M. gypseum* (Nannizzi, 1927, Stockdale, 1963) as well as in others. This places the species with a perfect state in the Class Ascomycetes. Using the hair-bait technique or the agar medium developed by Weitzman (see under laboratory procedures, p. 43), the ascigerous state may be developed in culture. *Nannizzia* is the perfect state for *Microsporum* species and *Arthroderma* is the perfect state for *Trichophyton* species. The perfect states of these organisms belong to the family Gymnoascaceae.

Microscopic Characteristics

In addition to variation in size, shape, thickness, and character of the wall of the macroconidia if present in the genus and species, the microconidia may be arranged along the sides of the hyphae or in grapelike clusters (en grappe), and be oval or pear-shaped. Other structures that may be present are: arthrospores, chlamydospores, nodular organs, pectinate bodies, racquet hyphae, and spirals. The macroconidia when present is the most important aid in identification of the organisms microscopically.

Colony Characteristics

The use of a standard medium, such as Sabouraud glucose agar, will be of value in the development of colonies similar to those described in reference books. The rate of growth, pattern, changes in color, on the surface and reverse side of the colony are observed for identification purposes. Variations within a species may occur, manifested by changes in color, rate of growth, or other observable changes. Some species very commonly develop white, cottony growths with sterile mycelium by mutation. This change, incorrectly known as "pleomorphism," appears on the surface of a normally growing colony, and may be readily located. If these sterile mycelial forms are isolated from lesions of patients, identification is difficult.

Physiological Requirements

Recent research has improved the procedures for identification of the dermatophytes on the basis of a better understanding of the nutritional requirements. Routine nutritional tests may be done to differentiate species of *Trichophyton* in addition to cultural studies and microscopic examination of the colony.

The dermatophytes grow at room temperature (25° C) at a pH of 6.8-7.0 although these fungi are tolerant of variation in pH and temperatures.

The use of cycloheximide (antifungal) and chloramphenicol (antibacterial), in the quantities recommended, in Sabouraud dextrose agar is useful in isolation of dermatophytes as saprophytic fungi and most bacteria are retarded.

The dermatophytes are able to utilize keratin, a substance found in epidermal tissues, but do not require it when growing in culture. Many keratinophilic fungi that do not produce disease in animals or man may be found in the soil.

DERMATOPHYTES

Imperfect Stage (Deuteromycete)	Perfect Stage (Ascomycete)
Microsporum Gruby, 1843 — attacks hair and skin.	
M. audouinii Gruby, 1843.	
M. canis Bodin, 1902	
M. cookei Ajello, 1959	*Nannizzia cajetani* Ajello, 1961
M. distortum di Menna and Marples, 1954	
M. ferrugineum Ota, 1922	
M. fulvum Uriburu 1909	*Nannizzia fulva* Stockdale, 1963
M. gypseum (Bodin) Guiart and Grigorakis, 1928	*Nannizzia incurvata* Stockdale, 1961
	Nannizzia gypsea (Nannizzi) Stockdale, 1963
M. nanum Fuentes, 1956	*Nannizzia obtusa* Dawson and Gentles, 1961
M. persicolor (Sabouraud) Guiget & Grigoraki, 1928	*Nannizzia persicolor* Stockdale, 1967
M. vanbreuseghemii Georg, Ajello, Friedman & Brinkman, 1962	*Nannizzia grubyia* Georg, Ajello, Friedman & Brinkman, 1962

Imperfect Stage (Deuteromycete)	Perfect Stage (Ascomycete)

Epidermophyton Sabouraud, 1910 — attacks skin and nails.

E. floccosum (Harz) Langeron and Milochevitch, 1930

Trichophyton Malmsten, 1845 — attacks skin, nails, and hair.

1. Ectothrix - invaded hair.

T. mentagrophytes (Robin) Blanchard, 1896	*Arthroderma benhamiae* Ajello and Cheng, 1967
T. equinum (Matruchot & Dassonville) Gedoelst, 1902	
T. rubrum (Castellani) Sabouraud, 1911	
T. verrucosum Bodin, 1902	

(Species not likely to be found in the United States)

T. gallinae (Megnin) Silva & Benham, 1952

T. megninii Blanchard, 1896

2. Ectothrix-endothrix - invaded hair

T. simii (Pinoy) Stockdale, Mackenzie & Austwick, 1965	*Arthroderma simii* Stockdale, Mackenzie & Austwick, 1965

3. Endothrix - invaded hair

T. tonsurans Malmsten, 1845

T. schoenleinii (Lebert) Langeron & Milochevitch, 1930 (Favus type)

T. violaceum Sabouraud, apud Bodin, 1902

T. gourvilii Catanei, 1933

T. soudanense Joyeux, 1912

T. yaoundei Cochet and Doby-Dubois, 1957

4. Hair not invaded

T. concentricum Blanchard, 1896

5. Saprophytic in Soil

T. ajelloi (Vanbreuseghem) Ajello, 1967	*Arthroderma uncinatum* Dawson & Gentles, 1961
T. georgiae Varsavsky & Ajello, 1964	*Arthroderma ciferrii* Varsavsky & Ajello, 1964
T. gloriae Ajello & Cheng, 1967	*Arthroderma gloriae* Ajello & Cheng, 1967
T. terrestre Durie & Frey, 1957	*Arthroderma quadrifidum* Dawson & Gentles, 1961

Imperfect Stage (Deuteromycete)	Perfect Stage (Ascomycete)
T. vanbreuseghemii Rioux, Jarry & Juminer, 1964	*Arthroderma gertleri* Bohme, 1967

Laboratory Suggestions for Study of the Dermatophytes

1. Young and older colonies of all the dermatophytes should be studied periodically to note changes, rates of growth, and morphological characteristics for differentiation of the individual species.

2. Slide cultures by the Riddell method or other methods, or direct mounts of the different species of the three genera should be made to study the microscopic characteristics (see methods, page 10).

3. Study procedures for obtaining materials from patients, and if ringworm cases are available, check the nail, skin, or hair material to see if it is positive. Then try several methods for isolation of the organism.

4. Use the Wood's light (see page 24) on the infected hairs to see the characteristic fluorescence. Check fluorescence of some organic substances.

5. Try isolating some unknowns that have been made from spore suspensions of known cultures in saline solution. If more than one organism is placed in the unknown, try to separate the organisms in pure culture.

6. When clinical cases of animal ringworm of the hair become available, such as *Microsporum canis* in a kitten, it is possible to keep the cases after death in the deep freeze for future use in class. Mosaic hairs on a kitten have remained viable nearly 17 years in the deep freeze. These can be readily used for microscopic study, and for isolation of the fungus in culture.

7. Isolate contaminated material from ringworm cases on media with and without actidione and antibacterial substances. Note the difference in the number of dermatophyte colonies isolated.

8. Grow the dermatophytes on several different media and note the difference in the morphological appearance of the colonies (see p. 36, 43).

9. Use visual aids such as film strips, kodachromes of cases, cultures and microscopic characteristics, and movies when available in the study of the dermatophytes.

10. Use of hair for isolation of dermatophytes from soil:

    a. Collect soil from areas with high organic content such as flower beds, barnyards, animal pathways, or other selected locations.

    b. Fill a petri dish approximately half full with the soil sample, which should be moistened with the addition of sterile distilled water containing 500 ug penicillin, 300 ug streptomycin, and 0.5 mg Actidione/ml (see p. 43).

    c. Scatter short pieces of sterilized human or horse hair over the surface of the soil and incubate at room temperature.

    d. Examine after one week for the development of hyphae on the surface of the hair. If fungal growth is present, place the hair on Sabouraud glucose agar with cycloheximide and chloramphenicol. Check the identification of the colony in 10 days or more. In some cases nonpathogenic keratinophilic fungi will be isolated.

    e. Check the hairs periodically for about 1 month for the development of cleistothecia or the perfect stage of some of the dermatophytes. Use Weitzman's medium for study of ascigerous state (see procedures, p. 43).

f. Some commonly isolated species are: *Microsporum gypseum, Trichophyton ajelloi,* and *Trichophyton terrestre.*

11. Set up the media for differentiation of the species of *Trichophyton* based on nutritional requirements (see procedures, p. 44).

12. The cellophane tape method may be used to pick up conidia and hyphae of dermatophytes from cultures or from ringworm cases for staining and slide mounts (see procedure, p. 10).

13. Use this soil-hair culture technique for the study of the perfect stage of the dermatophytes. Several of the dermatophytes will produce cleistothecia under suitable cultural conditions. The perfect stages of two genera *Nannizzia* and *Arthroderma,* related to the imperfect genera *Microsporum* and *Trichophyton* (see list of dermatophytes), can be grown on a soil-hair culture medium, or Weitzman's medium for study of the ascigerous state (see procedures, p. 43).

The two compatible strains for each species are inoculated on the surface of soil (sterilized or unsterilized) or agar medium in close proximity. Sterilized horse mane or tail hair, or child's hair, cut short, should be scattered over the surface of the soil. Other animal hair may be satisfactory, but human hair is unsatisfactory for the best production of cleistothecia (Dawson, Gentles and Brown, 1964). In approximately 3 to 4 weeks mature cleistothecia should be formed. Use same procedure for agar medium.

a. Example: Start with two stains of the heterothallic *Microsporum gypseum.* Inoculate these in close proximity on the soil-hair or agar medium and incubate at room temperature (24° C) for 3 to 4 weeks. Where the two strains unite, cleistothecia of *Nannizzia incurvata* will appear. Examine for presence of asci and ascospores, and peridial hyphae.

14. **Animal Inoculation:** This technique is useful for the laboratory study of the nature of the lesions developed by the organisms and to study immunity. Normally this technique is not used for identification of the dermatophytes. Guinea pigs, and sometimes mice, are used as the preferred animals for inoculation. Some species such as *Microsporum canis, M. gypseum,* or *Trichophyton mentagrophytes* may be established more readily in laboratory animals. The procedure according to Rivalier (1929) that is useful is as follows:

a. With a small surgical scissors cut the hair off an area about 2 cm² on the back of the guinea pig. The area may be abraded until reddened.

b. Prepare a heavy sporulation suspension of the fungus by grinding with some water or honey to make a paste.

c. Apply the paste to the area and rub in well.

d. In 7-10 days erythema and esquamation should be evident. Examine for the presence of the fungus.

e. If the hairs are not infected, check in 15 days.

f. Reisolate the organisms from the lesions.

NOTE: The animals usually will show no sign of the infection after 3 to 4 weeks.

Laboratory Diagnosis

Collection of Clinical Materials:

See directions under Preparation of Specimens in the section on Laboratory Procedure.

Laboratory Examination of Clinical Materials:

Examination of hairs, nails, or skin may give the first clue to a mycotic infection, but cultures must be made in order to determine the etiological agents.

Microscopic Structures

9 Racquet hyphae

10 Pectinate body

11 Nodular body

12 Favic chandelier

13 Chlamydospore

14 Coils

15 T. tonsurans Microconidia (borne singly)

16 T. mentagrophytes Microconidia (grapelike clusters)

17 T. terrestre conidia

18 T. rubrum Macroconidia

PLATE IV

Microsporum

Characteristics:

Microsporum consists of a number of species which attack hair and skin of animals and man. These fungi may cause ringworm of the scalp, beard, or body of man (tinea capitis, tinea barbae, and tinea corporis). The hyphae grow downward inside the hair shaft, forming a mosaic pattern around the outside of the hair shaft. Usually the metabolite produced by the fungus will fluoresce under Wood's light as a greenish color.

The organisms are usually isolated on Sabouraud glucose agar at room temperature with the addition of antibiotics. The colonies vary from moderately slow-growing, matted, and furrowed to fast-growing, powdery or velvety, and light tan, ferrugineous, yellowish to cinnamon in color. The reverse side of the colony may vary from reddish-brown, ferrugineous, yellowish to reddish-black.

The hyphae produce characteristic large, thin to thick, rough-walled, 3 to 15-celled, fusiform to obovate macroconidia. Two species, *M. gypseum* and *M. nanum,* have thin-walled macroconidia. Small one-celled microconidia are produced on short stalks or sessile on the hyphae; pectinate hyphae, racquet hyphae, nodular bodies, and chlamydospores may be present (see Plate IV).

Etiological Agents:

Microsporum audouinii is a common cause of tinea capitis, especially in children; *M. canis* is of animal origin, and occasionally causes tinea capitis or tinea corporis in man; *M. cookei* is a soil-inhabiting organism of little or no importance as an infective agent in man; *M. distortum* is a rare cause of tinea capitis; *M. ferrugineum* causes tinea capitis in children (of little importance in North America); *M. gypseum* is a soil-inhabiting fungus occasionally pathogenic in man and animals. This fungus usually causes an inflammatory reaction of the scalp known as kerion. Hairs may or may not fluoresce. *Microsporum nanum* is a rare cause of ringworm in man; *M. vanbreuseghemii* also is a rare cause of ringworm.

Laboratory Procedures

1. **Source of Infected Material:** Epilated hairs including the stubs should be placed in a sterile container or isolated directly on suitable media. Under Wood's light, the greenish fluorescent hairs may be readily plucked for laboratory diagnosis.

2. **Examination of Infected Material:**

   a. Place infected hair and skin if present on a slide containing a drop of 10% potassium hydroxide (KOH) and heat gently before examining. Lactophenol may also be used for hair specimens. Slides with infected hairs and lactophenol may be kept by sealing with fingernail polish or other types of cement.

   b. <u>Microscopically</u>, species of *Microsporum* form a dense spore sheath, mosaic in pattern around the hair shaft. Note that the growth of the fungus is located primarily around the outside of the hair. Hyphae may be seen in the epidermal cells of the skin in some cases.

3. **Cultures:** All of the species of *Microsporum* can be grown on Sabouraud glucose agar. The addition of actidone and chloromycetin may be desirable if the material is contaminated. At least two or three hair stubs should be placed on the medium and kept for at least two weeks. The use of other media, such as dermatophyte test medium and phyton peptone in a modification of Sabouraud agar is also desirable.

   a. *Microsporum audouinii,* Gruby, 1843

      (1) <u>Occurrence</u>:

         (a) <u>Man</u>: This species, originally endemic in Europe, now occurs in children, especially in North America, Europe and other parts of the world. Infected hairs fluoresce.

(b) <u>Animals</u>: *M. audouinii* has been reported on a dog and a capuchin monkey in the United States, and on a dog in England.

(2) <u>Colonies</u> on Sabouraud glucose agar develop slowly, forming a matted, velvety surface with straggly edges, and are light tan to brown in color. The reverse side is buff-salmon, to orange-brown (see Plate V). Growth on rice grains is poor.

(3) <u>Microscopically</u>, the macronidia are rare on Sabouraud agar. Macroconidia when found, are poorly formed and have thick, rough or smooth-walls. Some may be nearly spindle-shaped. Usually very irregular in shape (Fig. 41). The number of cells varies from a few to 8 or 9. Microconidia when present, are sessile or on short stalks along the hyphae, clavate and single-celled. Racquet hyphae, pectinate hyphae, nodular bodies and chlamydospores may be found (see Plate IV). Look for these structures in a direct mount or in a slide culture. Terminal chlamydospores are characteristic of this species.

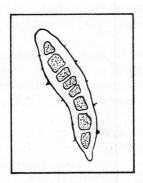

Figure 41

(4) <u>Special Comments</u>: Poor growth on rice helps to separate this species from *M. canis*. The addition of yeast extract to the medium may stimulate formation of macroconidia in some strains of *M. audouinii*. Infected hairs fluoresce.

b. *Microsporum canis,* Bodin, 1902

(1) <u>Occurrence</u>:

(a) <u>Man</u>: This fungus is the cause of tinea capitis and tinea corporis. The source of infection is usually from an animal (the organism is zoophilic). The disease is worldwide in distribution. Infected hairs usually fluoresce.

(b) <u>Animals</u>: *M. canis* has been isolated commonly from ringworm of cats and dogs, and less frequently from monkeys, horses, rabbits, and pigs.

(c) <u>Soil</u>: Reported from sand beaches in Hawaii and soil in Romania.

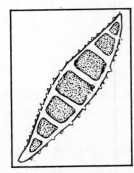

Figure 42

(2) <u>Colonies</u> on Sabouraud agar develop fairly rapidly, forming cottony or woolly mycelium, white to buff in color, and later becoming buff to brown in the center. The reverse side of the colony is yellow to orange-brown in color. The bright yellow color occurs when the colonies are 5 to 7 days old. This species grows well on rice grains (see Plate V).

(3) <u>Microscopically</u>, the macroconidia are characteristic of the species, i.e., they are numerous, large, many-celled, and spindle-shaped, with rough thick walls (see Plate II). The macroconidia are 8 to 20 by 40 to 150 μ in size and 6-15 celled (Plate V; Fig. 42). A few small, one-celled clavate to elongate microconidia may be found along the hyphae. Racquet hyphae, pectinate hyphae, nodular bodies, and chlamydospores may be seen.

(4) <u>Special Comments</u>: *M. canis* grows readily on rice grains (polished) while *M. audouinii* does not.

c. *Microsporum cookei*, Ajello, 1959

(1) <u>Occurrence</u>:

(a) <u>Man</u>: Skin infections have been reported in man.

(b) <u>Animals</u>: Although isolated from dogs, rats, and wild animals, no lesions were developed. Usually isolated from soil.

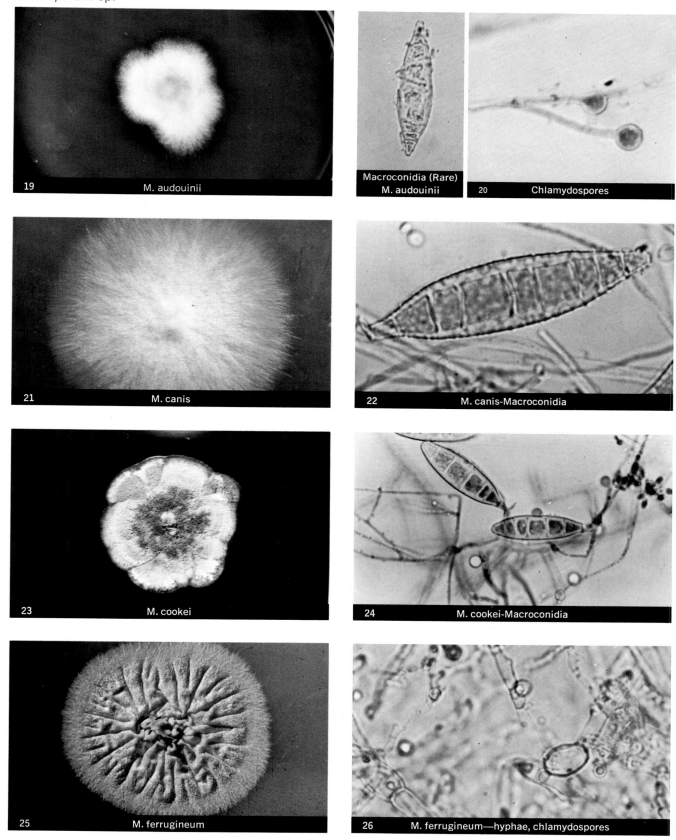

19   M. audouinii

Macroconidia (Rare)
M. audouinii   20   Chlamydospores

21   M. canis

22   M. canis-Macroconidia

23   M. cookei

24   M. cookei-Macroconidia

25   M. ferrugineum

26   M. ferrugineum—hyphae, chlamydospores

PLATE V

(2) <u>Colonies</u> on Sabouraud glucose agar develop rapidly, flat and spreading, with a rather powdery surface which is yellowish, buff or dark tan from the macroconidia mass. The organism resembles a mutant *M. gypseum* with dark pigments. Reverse side is deep purplish-red (see Plate V).

(3) <u>Microscopically</u>, the numerous macroconidia are oval to ellipsoidal, echinulate, with very thick walls (see Fig. 43). Microconidia are obovoid and abundant. The macroconidia are 31-50 by 10-15 μ on Sabouraud medium and similar to *M. gypseum* except for wall thickness (see Plate V).

(4) <u>Special Comments</u>: None.

(5) <u>Perfect Stage</u>: *Nannizzia cajetani*, Ajello, 1961. The ascomycetous state appears in some strains on hair. The cleistothecia are globose, pale buff to yellow color, 368-686 μ in diameter, peridial hyphae are slightly constricted, hyaline, septate, verticillately branched, and echinulate. Two kinds of appendages are present: elongated, slender tapered hyphae up to 480 μ long, and elongated, slender hyphae coiled into spirals. Asci are globose or ovate, 6-9 μ in diameter with 8 ascospores which are ovate, golden, smooth-walled, and 3-3.6 by 1.8 μ in size. Heterothallic.

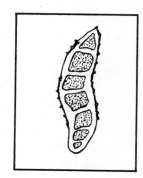

Figure 43

d. *Microsporum distortum,* di Menna and Marples, 1954

(1) <u>Occurrence</u>:

(a) <u>Man</u>: A few reports of tinea capitis in the United States, Australia, and New Zealand. Greenish flourescence in infected hairs.

(b) <u>Animals</u>: *M. distortum* has been reported in monkeys, dogs, horses, and pigs. Hairs fluoresce.

(2) <u>Colonies</u> on Sabouraud glucose agar develop fairly rapidly like *M. canis*, flat, velvety to fluffy, white to tan. The reverse side of the colony may have no color or be yellow to tan. Good growth on rice grains.

(3) <u>Microscopically</u>, macroconidia are like *M. canis*, being thick-walled with a rough surface, but bent and distorted (see Fig. 44). Clavate microconidia are sessile on the hyphae.

Figure 44

(4) <u>Special Comments</u>: *M. distortum* grows well on rice grains (polished) like *M. canis.*

e. *Microsporum ferrugineum,* Ota, 1922
(Synonym: *Trichophyton ferrugineum)*

(1) <u>Occurrence</u>:

(a) <u>Man</u>: This organism causes tinea capitis in children in Middle Europe, Asia, Russia, and Africa. Hairs fluoresce.

(b) <u>Animals</u>: Not reported.

(2) <u>Colonies</u> are rather slow-growing, heaped, with many deep furrows, glabrous and waxy, with a deep yellow to orange color (see Plate V). A white velvety cover may form over the colony. The colonies develop sectors readily with variations in color intensities, at times appearing as nonpigmented forms, resembling *T. verrucosum.*

(3) <u>Microscopically</u> the only structures seen are hyphae with chlamydospores. The small spored ectothrix type hair infection similar to *M. canis* is the basis for locating this species in the genus.

(4) <u>Special Comments</u>: No special nutritional requirements are necessary. Stock cultures should be maintained at room temperature.

f. *Microsporum gypseum,* (Bodin) Guiart and Grigorakis, 1928

    (1) <u>Occurrence</u>:

        (a) <u>Man</u>: This species, which is the cause of an inflammatory type tinea corporis or tinea capitis, is worldwide in distribution. Little or no fluorescence of infected hairs.

        (b) <u>Soil</u>: Geophilic in soil throughout world.

        (c) <u>Animals</u>: *M. gypseum* has been reported in dogs, horses, rabbits, squirrels, monkeys, cats, pigs, rats, and mice.

    (2) <u>Colonies</u> grow rapidly on Sabouraud agar, becoming powdery and buff to cinnamon-brown in color. Some strains may form white aerial mycelium at first and then become matted. In older colonies sterile hyphal growth (pleomorphism) develops rapidly as a cottony growth over the original powdery surface. Reverse side of colony is pale yellow to tan and occasionally red in some strains (Plate VI).

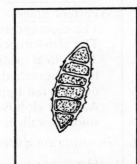

Figure 45

    (3) <u>Microscopically</u>, a slide culture or slide containing a portion of the colony will show numerous large, rough, thin-walled, ellipsoid, 3-9 celled, commonly 4-6 celled macroconidia, 8 to 12 by 30 to 50 μ in size, with echinulate walls (Plate VI, Fig. 45). Clavate microconidia are usually sessile on the hyphae.

    (4) <u>Special Comments</u>: None.

    (5) <u>Perfect Stages</u>: *Nannizzia incurvata,* Stockdale, 1961. The cleistothecia are globose, light buff or yellow buff and 350-650 μ in size when grown on hair. The peridial hyphae are asperulate septate (small constrictions), verticillately branched, and the branches curve out, then back. Some branches are spirally coiled at the apex. Asci are globose to ovate, 5-7 μ in size, with 8 smooth, lenticular ascospores, 2.8-3.5 by 1.5-2.0 μ in size. (Conidial form: *M. gypseum) Nannizzia gypsea* (Nannizzi) Stockdale, 1963. This is another perfect stage for *M. gypseum.* A third species, *M. fulvum,* although similar to *M. gypseum* in many respects, has been separated and linked to another perfect stage, *N. fulva.* For a more detailed discussion and description see Stockdale's article published in 1963.

g. *Microsporum nanum*, (Fuentes, Aboulafia and Vidal) Fuentes, 1956

    (1) <u>Occurrence</u>:

        (a) <u>Man</u>: First case in Cuba as tinea capitis. Rare in the United States.

        (b) <u>Animals</u>: Periodically causes tinea in pigs.

        (c) <u>Soil</u>: In United States, Mexico, Canada, and Australia.

    (2) <u>Colonies</u> resemble a mutant (pleomorphic) form of *M. gypseum.* The colony is white, cottony and spreading, becoming granular and buff-colored with the formation of many macroconidia. The reverse side of the colony is frequently red to brown (Plate VI).

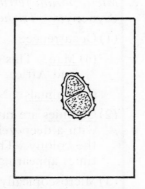

Figure 46

    (3) <u>Microscopically</u>, the characteristic macroconidia are small, pear-shaped, or clavate, rather thin-walled, usually verrucose; the spore is 2- or 3-celled, 12-18 by 4-7.5 μ in size (Plate VI; Fig. 46). Numerous microconidia may be formed on hair and soil cultures, while only a few are formed on Sabouraud agar. The hair filaments are perforated in vitro. Ectothrix type (sparse) on animals or humans, with little or no fluorescence.

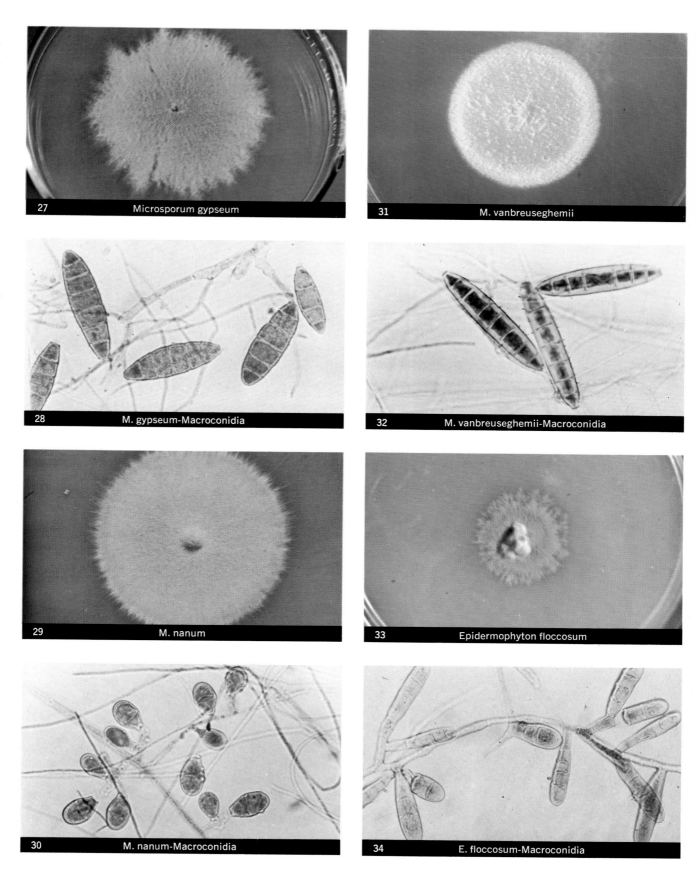

27   Microsporum gypseum

31   M. vanbreuseghemii

28   M. gypseum-Macroconidia

32   M. vanbreuseghemii-Macroconidia

29   M. nanum

33   Epidermophyton floccosum

30   M. nanum-Macroconidia

34   E. floccosum-Macroconidia

PLATE VI

(4) <u>Special Comments</u>: None.

(5) <u>Perfect Stage</u>: *Nannizzia obtusa,* Dawson and Gentles, 1961. The cleistothecia are globose, 250-450 μ in diameter, with pale yellow peridial hyphae. Peridial hyphae pale yellow, hyaline, septate, branched dichotomously, at obtuse angle from main hypha, cells thick-walled, echinulate, cylindrical, about 13 by 4-7 μ, 1-2 slight constrictions. Appendages are septate, smooth-walled, with lateral or terminal tightly coiled spirals. Asci subglobose, evanescent, 5.5 by 5-6 μ in size. Eight ascospores, usually smooth, lenticular, 2.7-3.2 by 1.2-2 μ in size, and yellowish.

h. *Microsporum vanbreuseghemii,* Georg, Ajello, Friedman, & Brinkman, 1962

  (1) <u>Occurrence</u>:

    (a) <u>Man</u>: A rare ringworm infection reported in the United States, also in Europe.

    (b) <u>Animals</u>: Reported in a dog and a squirrel in the United States.

  (2) <u>Colonies</u> are fast-spreading, flat, surface powdery or downy, creamy-yellow to pink in color. The reverse side of the colony is colorless to yellow. Variants or pleomorphism develops readily (Plate VI).

  (3) <u>Microscopically</u>, the numerous macroconidia are cylindro-fusiform, 7-10 septations, thick-walled with a rough surface (Plate VI; Fig. 47). These rough or echinulate macroconidia are 58.8-61.7 by 10.4-10.6 μ in size. Microconidia may be abundant, pyriform to obovate in shape.

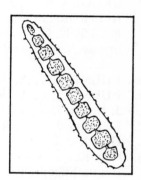

Figure 47

  (4) <u>Special Comments</u>: This species differs from *T. ajelloi* by the lack of a purple pigment, readily infects guinea pigs, and has echinulate macroconidia. Little or no fluorescence of infected hairs.

  (5) <u>Perfect Stage</u>: *Nannizzia grubyia,* Georg, Ajello, Friedman and Brinkman, 1962. The cleistothecia are globose, white to pale buff, and 150-600 μ in diameter. The peridial hyphae are hyaline, septate, branched dichotomously and branched uncinately usually curving away from main hyphae. Cells thick-walled, echinulate, phalangiform, 2-7.5 μ in diameter. Spirals terminal on peridial hyphae. Asci globose, evanescent, 4.8-6.0 μ in size with 8 hyaline, smooth-walled, yellow, oval ascospores, 2.4 by 3.0 μ in size. Heterothallic.

4. **Animal Inoculation:** *M. gypseum* and *M. canis* and some of the other species will infect kittens, puppies, young rabbits, and other young laboratory animals. In 3 to 5 days after inoculation, a severe inflammatory reaction develops, and later a heavy crust. Some of the hair may become involved and drop out as in alopecia. After a month or more the laboratory animals usually recover spontaneously. If laboratory animals are inoculated, observe the course of the infection.

<u>Questions:</u>

1. What are the important macroscopic and microscopic characteristics used to distinguish the species of the genus *Microsporum*? Select the key characteristics for each species and learn to recognize them.

2. Is it possible to distinguish the species of *Microsporum* causing a tinea capitis case by microscopic examination of an infected hair? Explain.

3. Of what value is the Wood's light in the laboratory identification of *Microsporum* sp.? Is there any difference in fluorescence between species of *Microsporum?*

4. What is the value to the physician of specific identification of the fungus in cases of tinea capitis?

Selected References

1. AJELLO, L. 1956. Soil as a natural reservoir for human pathogenic fungi. Science. 123:876.
2. AJELLO, L. 1959. A new *Microsporum* and its occurrence on man and animals. Mycologia. 51:69.
3. AJELLO, L. 1961. The ascigerous state of *Microsporum cookei.* Sabouraudia 1:173.
4. AJELLO, L. 1968. A taxonomic review of the dermatophytes and related species. Sabouraudia 6:147.
5. AJELLO, L., E. Varsavsky, O. J. Ginther and G. Bubash. 1964. The natural history of *Microsporum nanum.* Mycologia 56:873.
6. ALTERAS, I., and R. Evolceanu. 1969. First isolation of *Microsporum racemosum* Dante Borelli 1965 from Romanian soil (new data on its pathogenic properties). Mykosen. 12:223.
7. BROCK, J. M. 1961. *Microsporum nanum:* A cause of tinea capitis. Arch. Dermat. 84:504.
8. BROOKS, B. E., J. H. Alli and C. C. Campbell. 1959. Isolation of *Microsporum distortum* from a human case. J. Invest. Dermat. 33:23.
9. DAWSON, C. O. and J. C. Gentles. 1961. The perfect stages of *Keratinomyces ajelloi* Vanbreuseghem, *Trichophyton terrestre* Durie and Frey, *Microsporum nanum* Fuentes. Sabouraudia. 1:49.
10. FUENTES, C. A. 1956. A new species of *Microsporum.* Mycologia. 43:613.
11. FUENTES, C. A., R. Aboulafia and R. J. Vidal. 1954. A dwarf form of *Microsporum gypseum.* J. Invest. Derm. 23:51.
12. GEORG, L. K. 1960. Animal ringworm in public health. Diagnosis and nature. U.S. Dept. of Health, Education and Welfare, Communicable Disease Center, Atlanta.
13. GEORG, L. K., L. Ajello, L. Friedman and S. A. Brinkman. 1962. A new species of *Microsporum* pathogenic to man and animals. Sabouraudia 1:189.
14. GIBLETT, E. R. and B. S. Henry. 1950. Physiological studies on the genus *Microsporum.* J. Invest. Derm. 14:377.
15. GORDON, M. A. 1953. The occurrence of the dermatophyte *Microsporum gypseum,* as a saprophyte in soil. J. Invest. Derm. 20:201.
16. HAZEN, E. L. 1947. *Microsporum audouini:* The effect of yeast extract thiamine, pyridoxine, and *Bacillus Weidmaniensis* on the colony characteristics and macroconidial formation. Mycologia 39:200.
17. HAZEN, E. L. 1957. Effect of temperature and nutrition upon macroconidial formation of *Microsporum audouini.* Mycologia 49:11.
18. KAPLAN, W., L. K. Georg, L. Hendricks and R. A. Leeper. 1954. Isolation of *Microsporum distortum* from animals in the United States. J. Invest. Derm. 28:449.
19. EVOLCEANU, R. and I. Alteras. 1967. Isolierung von *Microsporum canis* aus Bodenproben in Rumanien (Bukarest). Mykosen 10:243.
20. LA TOUCHE, C. J. 1955. Onychomycosis in cats infected by *Microsporum canis* Bodin. Vet. Rec. 67:578.
21. KISHIMOTO, R. A. and G. E. Baker. 1969. Pathogenic and potentially pathogenic fungi isolated from beach sands and selected soils of Oahu, Hawaii. Mycologia 61:537.
22. LEIGHTON, T. J. and J. J. Stock. 1969. Heat-induced macroconidia germination in *Microsporum gypseum.* Appl. Microbiol. 17:473.
23. LOEWENTHAL, K. 1950. Effect of yeast extract on *Microsporum audouini* and *Microsporum canis.* Arch. Derm. and Syph. 62:265.
24. LUNDELL, E. 1969. *Microsporum cookei* Ajello in an eczematous skin lesion. Mykosen 12:123.
25. ORR, G. F. 1969. Keratinophilic fungi isolated from soils by a modified hair bait technique. Sabouraudia 7:129.
26. PADHYE, A. A. 1969. Cellophane mounts of ascigerous states of dermatophytes and other keratinophilic fungi. Mycologia 60:1242.

27. REISS, F., L. Caroline and L. Leonard. 1954. Experimental *Microsporum lanosum* infection in dogs, cats, and rabbits. I. Observations on the course of the primary infection. Trans. N. Y. Acad. Sci. Ser. II. 16(5):277.

28. SIK, G. 1965. Microsporia on the smooth skin, caused by *Microsporum cookei* Ajello 1959. Derm. Vener. (Sofia). 4:6.

29. STOCKDALE, P. M. 1961. *Nannizzia incurvata*, gen. nov., sp. nov. a perfect state of *Microsporum gypseum*. Sabouraudia. 1:41.

30. STOCKDALE, P. M. 1963. The *Microsporum gypseum* Complex *(Nannizzia incurvata* Stockd., *N. gypsea* (Nann.) comb. nov., *N. fulva* sp. nov.) Sabouraudia 3:114.

31. STOCKDALE, P. M. 1967. *Nannizzia persicolor* sp. nov., the perfect state of *Trichophyton persicolor* Sabouraud. Sabouraudia 5:355.

32. WHITTLE, C. H. 1954. A small epidemic of *Microsporum gypseum* ringworm in a plant nursery. Brit. J. Derm. 66:353.

33. WOLF, F. T., E. A. Jones and H. A. Nathan. 1958. Fluorescent pigment of *Microsporum*. Nature, London 182:475.

Epidermophyton

Characteristics:

Epidermophyton consists of a single species that attacks the skin and nails. This organism is a common cause of tinea cruris and tinea pedis. It may cause epidemics in institutions, camps, and other group gatherings.

Etiological Agent:

Epidermophyton floccosum (Harz) Langeron and Milochevitch, 1930, is the only species placed in this genus. In addition to causing tinea cruris and tinea pedis, the nail may be invaded, resulting in tinea unguium.

Occurrence:

1. **Man:** *E. floccosum* is found throughout the world, having a higher rate of occurrence in the tropics.

2. **Animals:** No reported domestic animal cases.

Laboratory Procedures

1. **Source of Infected Material:** Skin scrapings or pieces of nail should be placed in a sterile container or isolated directly on suitable media.

2. **Examination of Infected Material:**

   a. Place infected skin or pieces of nail on a slide containing a drop of 10% to 20% potassium hydroxide and add a cover glass. Heat gently to clear and soften the material.

   b. Semi-permanent Mount: Although there are a number of methods for staining hairs and scales for permanent slides, the following method has been satisfactory for skin or nail material if the washing procedure is carefully followed. With reasonable care after the slides are sealed with fingernail polish, the slides should last for a long period of time.

   Procedure:

   (1) Place the material (skin or nail) in a small glass container with 10% to 20% KOH (thin flakes of skin for 5 minutes and small pieces of nail for 20 minutes or more).

   (2) The digested material is removed from the KOH solution by decanting.

   (3) Wash thoroughly with water two or three times for 5 to 10 minutes each time.

   (4) Wash two or three more times with 1% lactic acid or acetic acid to neutralize the material.

   (5) Mount small pieces of the material in lactophenol and seal cover glass with fingernail polish.

   c. Microscopically, the fungus appears in the material as septate, branching mycelial strands identical in appearance with those that may be found in *Microsporum* skin infections. The threadlike hyphae of the fungus may be seen under the low power of the microscope, but more details of the hyphae and arthrospores may be seen under higher magnification (Plate I, Fig. 8).

   Precautions:

   (1) Do not mistake fat globules or air bubbles for arthrospores or the crystals of KOH that give a mosaic pattern for the branching mycelium.

   (2) At least two or more preparations of randomly selected material should be made before a negative microscopic finding is reported. A confirmatory culture should be made for additional information when desirable.

3. **Cultures:** The fungus grows readily at room temperature on Sabouraud glucose agar with the addition of chloromycetin and actidione to prevent bacterial contamination and overgrowth by saprophytic molds. Three or four pieces of infected material should be placed on the agar medium.

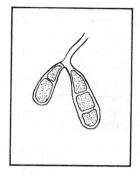

Figure 48

a. <u>Colonies</u> develop fairly rapidly with a velvety to powdery surface, greenish-yellow color, and a cottony center. The reverse side of the colony is yellow to tan in color. The greenish-yellow colonies usually develop numerous radiating furrows. In several weeks some strains become covered with the pleomorphic form which is cottony with mostly white, sterile aerial mycelium (see Plate VI). Study the rate of growth.

b. <u>Microscopically</u>, many large clavate, smooth, thin-walled, 2- to 6-celled macroconidia, 7 to 12 by 20 to 40 μ in size, single or in clusters. No microconidia are produced. Chlamydospores, racquet hyphae, and nodular bodies may be present (see Plate IV). Occasionally spirals may be found. Observe these on a slide or a slide culture (Plate VI; Fig. 48).

4. **Special Comments:** Stock cultures may be difficult to maintain, as colonies are pleomorphic and low temperature is not favorable.

5. **Animal Inoculation:** Laboratory animals are not successfully infected.

Questions:

1. Distinguish the genus *Epidermophyton* from *Microsporum.*

2. Is it possible to distinguish mycelium of *Epidermophyton, Microsporum,* and *Trichophyton* in infected skin or nail material?

Selected References

1. AJELLO, L. and M. E. Getz. 1954. Recovery of dermatophytes from shoes and shower stalls. J. Invest. Derm. 22:17.
2. CASTELLANI, A. 1910. Observations on new species of *Epidermophyton* found in tinea cruris. Brit. J. Derm. 22:147.
3. DUPERRAT, B., Badillet, G. and N. D. Toan. 1968. Fréquence d'*Epidermophyton floccosum* dans la région Parisienne. (A propos d'une épidémie d'épidermophytie chez de jeunes handicapés physiques.). Annls. Derm. Syph. 95:39.
4. LLOYD, K. M. and J. E. Greer. 1961. Two clinical variations in *Epidermophyton* infections. Archs. Derm. 84:2.
5. Mc CORMACK, P. and R. W. Benham. 1952. An unusual finding in *Epidermophyton floccosum.* J. Invest. Derm. 19:315.
6. WEIDMAN, F. D. 1926. Laboratory aspects of epidermophytosis. Arch. Derm. and Syph. 15:415.

Trichophyton

Characteristics:

Trichophyton consists of a large number of species which attack the skin, nails, and hair, resulting in a wide variety of symptoms, depending upon the species and the location of the infection. Infected hairs have arthrospores in parallel rows on the outside of the shaft (ectothrix type) or in parallel rows inside the shaft (endothrix type). This genus is the most likely cause of tinea pedis and tinea unguium in humans. Other types of ringworm in adults and children also may be due to species in this genus. The clinical symptoms vary considerably for this group of organisms so that laboratory identification is necessary for final diagnosis. Usually no fluorescence occurs in hairs infected by *Trichophyton* sp.

Most of the *Trichophyton* species may be isolated on Sabouraud glucose agar at room temperature. The addition of antibacterial substances and antifungal substances for inhibiting saprophytes is desirable. Specific media may be needed for species identification.

<u>Colonies</u> of this genus may appear cottony to velvety, granular to powdery, raised, or wrinkled and folded with a velvety to waxy surface. Pigmentation varies from white, pink, red, purple, violet, yellow, or orange to brown.

<u>Microscopically</u> some species have numerous microconidia that are small, single-celled, spherical, clavate, or pyriform in shape, and borne singly on the sides of hyphae (en thyrse) or in grapelike clusters (en grappe). Macroconidia which are rare or lacking in some species appear as long, thin-walled, many-celled clavate to fusiform structures, 20-50 by 4-8 μ in size. Racquet hyphae, nodular bodies, coiled hyphae and chlamydospores may be present.

Etiological Agents:

In 1968 there were 20 species that appeared distinct (Ajello, 1968). Ajello (1968) transferred the genus *Keratinomyces* to *Trichophyton* along with the new combinations *T. ajelloi* and *T. longifusus*. A new species was described, *T. gloriae* by Ajello and Cheng (1967). There are six species that invade the hair to produce an ectothrix type infection. The following four are common in the United States: *Trichophyton mentagrophytes* (Robin) Blanchard, 1896; *T. equinum* (Matruchot and Dassonville) Gedoelst, 1902; *T. rubrum* (Castellani) Sabouraud, 1911; and *T. verrucosum* Bodin, 1902. The two species not likely to be reported in the United States are: *T. gallinae* (Megnin) Silva and Benham, 1952; and *T. megninii* Blanchard, 1896.

In the six species which produce an ectothrix type hair infection, the arthrospores are formed on the outside of the hair shaft. The following seven species have an endothrix type hair invasion with the hyphae breaking up into arthrospores inside the hair shaft, except that *T. schoenleinii* is of the "favic type" with less breaking up of hyphae into arthrospores. Three occur in the United States: *T. tonsurans* Malmsten, 1945; *T. schoenleinii* (Lebert) Langeron and Milochevitch, 1930; and *T. violaceum* Bodin, 1902. The other four endothrix species not likely to occur in the United States are: *T. gourvillii* Catanei, 1933; *T. simii* (Pinoy) Stockdale, Mackenzie and Austwick, 1965; *T. soudanense* Joyeux, 1912; and *T. yaoundei* Cochet and Doby-Dubois, 1957. The hair is not invaded in the following species: *T. concentricum* Blanchard, 1896. The following five have been isolated as saprophytes from soil: *T. georgii* Varsavsky and Ajello, 1964 (Perfect Stage: *Arthroderma ciferrii* Varsavsky and Ajello, 1964); *T. terrestre* Durie and Frey 1957 (Perfect Stage: *Arthroderma quadrifidum* Dawson and Gentles, 1961); *T. ajelloi* (Vanbreuseghem) Ajello, 1967 (Perfect Stage: *Arthroderma uncinatum* Dawson and Gentles, 1961); *T. gloriae* Ajello and Cheng, 1967 (Perfect Stage: *Arthroderma gloriae* Ajello and Cheng, 1967); *T. vanbreuseghemii* Rioux, Jarry and Juminer, 1964 (*Arthroderma gertleri* Bohme, 1967).

Laboratory Procedures

1. **Source of Infected Materials:** Scrapings of the skin and shavings of the nail should be collected from the active border of the lesions where the fungus is more likely to be found. Infected hairs should be epilated. The specimens should be collected in a sterile container or paper packets or isolated directly on the proper medium.

2. **Examination of Infected Material:**

   a. Place the infected hair, skin, or nail on a slide with 10% potassium hydroxide and add a cover glass. Heat gently to clear and soften the material. In case hair is put in lactophenol, the slide may be sealed and kept for future reference. Positive skin or nail material may be preserved by the semi-permanent mount method (see *Epidermophyton*). The nail and skin material also may be stained with periodic acid-Schiff stain (see stain procedures, page 30). The addition of blue-black ink to the potassium hydroxide will aid in differentiation of the fungus material. The DMSO medium (see procedure, page 29) may be used.

   b. Microscopically, these fungi appear as septate, branching mycelial strands similar to *Microsporum* and *Epidermophyton* mycelial strands in the skin or nail. Older hyphae may have arthrospores. Be sure to differentiate any artefacts from the fungus hyphae in the determination of positive material. Let slide stand until artefacts appear and compare with hyphae, if the potassium hydroxide is used.

   Microscopically, the infected hairs will show rows of arthrospores inside the hair shaft (endothrix type) or outside the hair shaft (ectothrix type). *Trichophyton schoenleinii* and *T. violaceum* may show cup-shaped crusts (scutula) at the base of the hair shaft. The former also will have air spaces in the areas left by the degenerate hyphae and few or no arthrospores inside the hair shaft.

3. **Cultures:** All of the species of *Trichophyton* can be grown at room temperature; *T. verrucosum* does better with the addition of yeast extract to Sabouraud glucose agar. At least two or three pieces of skin, nail, or hair stubs should be placed on the agar medium and kept for two weeks or more before considering negative. The addition of cycloheximide and chloramphenicol to the medium is desirable for the isolation of these species from clinical materials. Other media such as dermatophyte test medium may be used. See media for preparation.

4. **Nutritional Tests for the Differentiation of *Trichophyton* Species:**

   a. Procedures: Acid-cleaned glassware should be used for the nutritional tests. The stock media consists of casein or ammonium nitrate agar, while the test media have the addition of thiamine, inositol, nicotinic acid, or histidine added singly or in combination to one of the above basal media. For preparation of the media, see technique section. The inoculum may be taken from cultures grown on any of the usual media. It is important to take a very small uniform fragment for each transfer to avoid a carry-over of the nonvitamin free medium.

   In reading the results on Table II for the nutritional patterns, a 4+ indicates maximum growth for the series of test tubes when comparing with the colony growth of other tubes. A ± indicates a trace of submerged growth around the inoculum. The use of these media are especially helpful in differentiation of *T. equinum* and *T. mentagrophytes, T. tonsurans* from *T. mentagrophytes, T. gallinae* from *T. megninii*, and *T. verrucosum* from some strains of *T. schoenleinii*.

TABLE II
Nutritional Patterns for *Trichophyton**

Species	Test Media	
	Casein	Casein + Nicotinic Acid
T. equinum	0	4+
T. mentagrophytes	4+	4+
	Casein	Casein + Thiamine
T. mentagrophytes	4+	4+
T. rubrum	4+	4+
T. tonsurans	± to 1+	4+
T. violaceum	±	4+
M. ferrugineum	4+	4+
	NH_4NO_3	NH_4NO_3 + Histidine
T. gallinae	4+	4+
T. megninii	0	4+

Species		Casein	Casein + Inositol	Casein + Thiamine	Casein + Thiamine & Inositol
*T. schoenleinii***		4+	4+	4+	4+
*T. verrucosum***	84%	0	±	0	4+
	16%	0	0	4+	4+
*T. concentricum***	50%	4+	4+	4+	4+
	50%	2+	2+	4+	4+

*Use two test tubes, room temperature, 7-10 days.
**Use four tubes, 37° C, 7-14 days.

Trichophyton sp—colonies
Ectothrix type hair invasion (35-42)

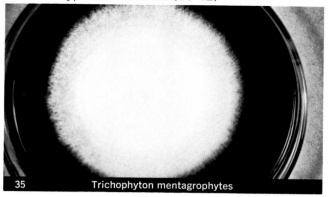

35   **Trichophyton mentagrophytes**

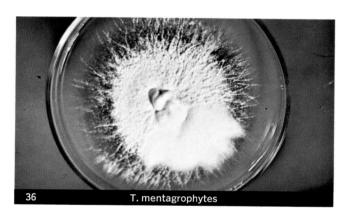

36   **T. mentagrophytes**

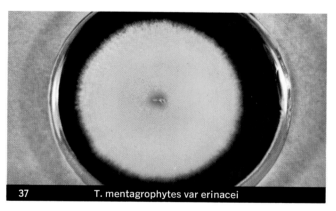

37   **T. mentagrophytes var erinacei**

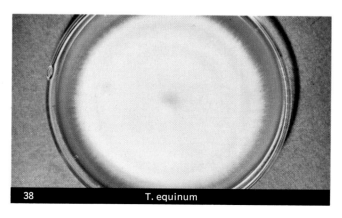

38   **T. equinum**

PLATE VII

1. Ectothrix Hair Invasion

A. *Trichophyton mentagrophytes* (Robin) Blanchard, 1896

    1. **Occurrence:**

        (a) <u>Man</u>: This species is a common cause of an inflammatory type ringworm on the feet (athlete's foot) or tinea pedis, hands, smooth skin area (tinea corporis) and nails (tinea unguium). It is also on the beard (tinea barbae) and scalp (tinea capitis). Infections occur throughout the world.

        (b) <u>Animals</u>: This organism may cause ringworm in cattle, horses, dogs, cats, sheep, pigs, rabbits, squirrels, monkeys, chinchillas, silver foxes, laboratory rats, mice, and at times in other animals.

    2. **Colonies** develop rather rapidly, forming a powdery to granular surface, light buff to rose-tan in color. On subsequent transfers or in older colonies a fluffy, cottony, white mycelium appears. The reverse side of the colony is light buff to deep wine or brown (see Plate VII).

    3. **Microscopically,** a lactophenol slide mount of a powdery or granular culture will show numerous microconidia singly and in clusters along the hyphae (en grappe). The microconidia are round, thin-walled, one-celled. Characteristic spirals, nodular bodies, chlamydospores and racquet hyphae may be present. The cottony colonial forms should have fewer conidia and other structures present. The macroconidia may be rare or numerous in different strains (Fig. 49), clavate to variable in shape, 3 to 5-celled, thin-walled, and 4-7 by 20-50 μ in size. For microconidia and other structures on hyphae, see Plate IV.

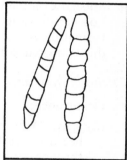

Figure 49

    4. **Special Comments:** No special nutrients needed. On autoclaved hair, *T. mentagrophytes* will perforate it and *T. rubrum* will not. On cornmeal agar the red strains of this species produce no color. On potato dextrose agar this species produces no color while *T. rubrum* produces a deep rose red color. Urease test is positive in 7 days.

    6. **Perfect Stage:** *Arthroderma benhamiae* Ajello and Cheng, 1967. Cleistothecia globose, 400-500 μ in diameter, white. Peridial hyphae hyaline, interwoven, asperulate, dumbbell-shaped with spiral appendages. Asci globose, thin-walled, hyaline, evanescent, with 8 ascospores. Heterothallic.

B. *Trichophyton equinum* (Matruchot & Dassonville) Gedoelst, 1902

    1. **Occurrence:**

        (a) <u>Man</u>: Usually does not occur in man.

        (b) <u>Animals</u>: Commonly a cause of ringworm in horses, occasionally in dogs. Worldwide except Australia and Africa.

    2. **Colonies** grow rapidly, flat, developing folds when older, surface white, cottony with yellow color in the edge around the new growth. Later the colony becomes velvety and cream-tan in color. The reverse side of the colony is bright yellow at first, becoming dark pink to brown in time. Nicotinic acid (niacin) is required for growth (see Plate VII).

    3. **Microscopically,** a few or many thin elongate to pyriform microconidia (rarely macroconidia) of the *T. mentagrophytes* type are produced. Nodular bodies and other structures may be present.

4. **Special Comments:** Nicotinic acid is a special nutritional requirement for this fungus, and horse hair, not human hair, must be used for culture in vitro.

C. *Trichophyton rubrum* (Castellani) Sabouraud, 1911

   1. **Occurrence:**

      (a) <u>Man</u>: A frequent cause of tinea corporis, tinea pedis, tinea cruris, and tinea unguium. Lesions with marked reddened margins and central clearings. Distributed throughout the world.

      (b) <u>Animals</u>: Rare in animals, but reported in a dog, a cat, a rabbit, a monkey, and a sheep. Also found in two cows.

   2. **Colonies** that are primary isolates are cottony and white, and later become velvety. The reverse side of the colony develops reddish to rose-purple pigmentation which may appear on the top surface of marginal hyphae (see Plate VIII).

   3. **Microscopically,** numerous clavate microconidia are in clusters and along edges of the hyphae on slides made from primary cultures, or slide cultures. Usually few macroconidia, chlamydospores, racquet hyphae, and nodular bodies are produced in primary cultures. Numerous long, thin-walled, 3-8 celled macroconidia are formed in cultures on heart infusion tryptose agar. Observe as many of these structures as possible under the microscope (see Plate IV).

   4. **Special Comments:** No special nutrients are needed. On autoclaved hair, *T. rubrum* will not perforate it in vitro. On potato dextrose agar and cornmeal dextrose agar the pigment formation for some strains is very marked for this species while *T. mentagrophytes* produces no red color. Urease test is negative in 7 days.

D. *Trichophyton verrucosum* Bodin, 1902

   1. **Occurrence:**

      (a) <u>Man</u>: A highly inflammatory infection involving the areas of the scalp (tinea capitis), beard (tinea barbae), and exposed areas of the body (tinea corporis). This species occurs throughout the world.

      (b) <u>Animals</u>: This species is most likely to be the cause of ringworm in cattle. Other animals include: donkey, dog, goat, sheep, and horse.

   2. **Colonies** develop better on enriched media such as Sabouraud glucose agar plus yeast extract or heart infusion tryptose agar with 1 mg of thiamine per 100 ml of melted medium. The colonies are slow growing, heaped, deeply folded, glabrous and waxy or with a fine white velvety surface. Colors vary in isolations from white to bright yellow. Study the growth rate of this species and compare with other *Trichophyton* species. Some strains require both thiamine and inositol for growth. More rapid growth occurs at 37° C (see Plate VIII).

   3. **Microscopically,** only chlamydospores are seen in the hyphae on Sabouraud dextrose agar. On media enriched with thiamine, microconidia are usually produced, and on rare occasions 3- to 5-celled macroconidia, varying in size and shape, may be seen.

   4. **Special Comments:** Special nutrients are needed — thiamine and for many strains, inositol. There are three variants in colonies known as "album," "discoides" and "ochraceum." Stock cultures should be kept at room temperature and not in the refrigerator.

E. *Trichophyton gallinae* (Megnin) Silva and Benham, 1952

   1. **Occurrence:**

      (a) <u>Man</u>: Very rare in man — apparently only two cases reported in children.

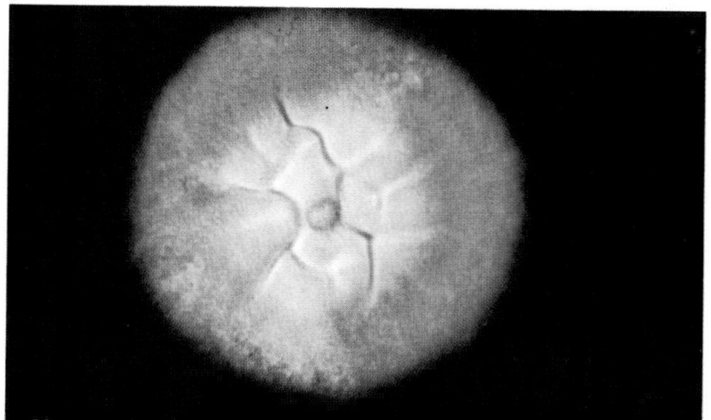

T. rubrum

40

T. megninii

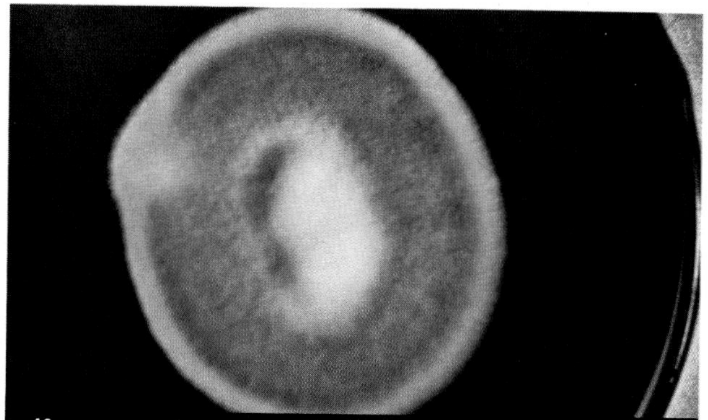

42

T. verrucosum

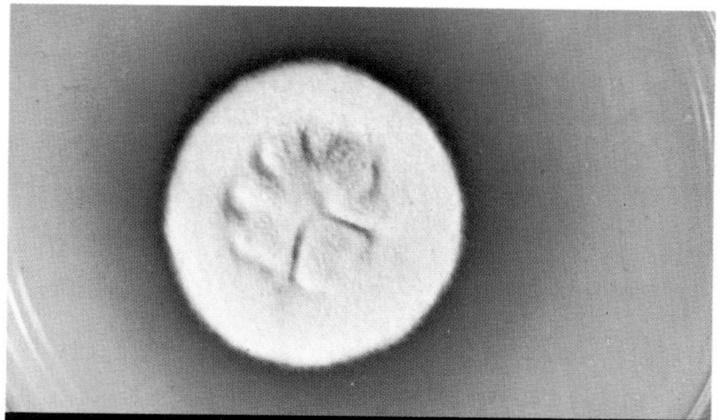

39

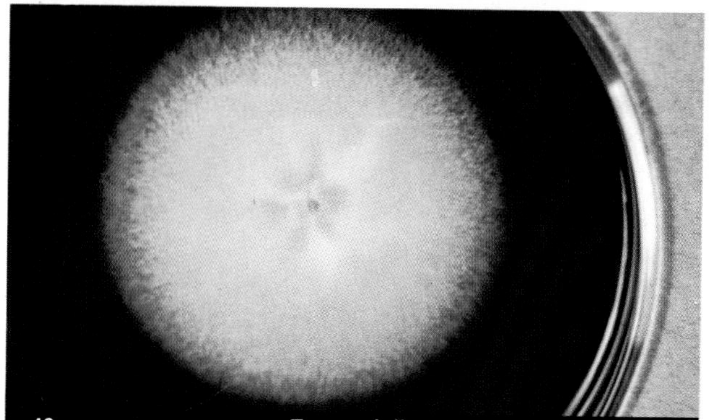

T. gallinae

41

PLATE VIII

(b) Animals: A cause of ringworm or favus in chickens throughout the world. Also reported in cat, mouse, and dog.

2. **Colonies** are moderately fast-growing, at first flat, then heaped with radial folds. Older folds may show color. Edges of colonies may be irregular. A deep strawberry-red color diffuses throughout the medium, later becoming deep red. Note the changes as the colony gets older. The surface becomes light pink and the entire medium is deep red (see Plate VIII).

3. **Microscopically,** a few small, pyriform to clavate microconidia may be seen, borne singly along the hyphae or in clusters. Macroconidia may be numerous, and are clavate, 2- to 10-celled, and smooth-walled. The addition of thiamine or yeast extract may increase sporulation.

4. **Special Comments:** No special nutritional needs.

F. *Trichophyton megninii* Blanchard, 1896

1. **Occurrence:**

(a) Man: This fungus is the primary cause of tinea barbae and occasionally the cause of tinea corporis and tinea capitis in Europe and Africa.

(b) Animals: No known infections.

2. **Colonies** are slow-growing, cottony to velvety and white at first, becoming pink later. A nondiffusible rose to red pigment develops on the reverse side. The addition of L-histidine to a special medium or the use of trypticase dextrose agar stimulates growth. Compare with *T. gallinae* (see Plate VIII).

3. **Microscopically,** numerous, small, pyriform to clavate microconidia may be seen singly or in clusters along the hyphae. Macroconidia, which are rare, develop as clavate, 2- to 10-celled, with thin, smooth walls.

4. **Special Comments:** Special nutrients needed. This species requires L-histidine for growth.

2. Ecto-Endothrix Hair Invasion

A. *Trichophyton simii* (Pinoy) Stockdale, Mackenzie, and Austwick, 1965

1. **Occurrence:**

(a) Man: Several cases from contact with animals. Hair invasion of the ecto-endothrix type.

(b) Animals: Ringworm infection, originating in or from India, has been found in monkeys, poultry and a dog.

(c) Soil: Occurs as a saprophyte.

2. **Colonies** are fast-growing, 75-84 mm. in diameter in 14 days at 25° C., with a conical, velvety, umbo center, finely granular. The surface is white to pale buff or rosy buff, and the reverse side is colorless at first, later vinaceous. In 3 or 4 weeks the vinaceous color may diffuse into the medium and onto the surface, if on 2.5% malt extract agar. On glucose peptone agar the surface is pale buff with the reverse color straw to salmon.

3. **Microscopically,** there are numerous smooth-walled, cylindrical to fusiform macroconidia on complexly branched hyphae with 4 to 7 (sometimes up to 10) septa. Microconidia are rare at first, more numerous later, clavate to pyriform with a narrow base. Spirals may be present.

4. **Special Comments:** No special nutrients needed. Colonies grow more rapidly than *T. mentagrophytes,* are thinner and more granular. On malt extract agar *A. simii* produces a vina-

ceous color while *T. mentagrophytes* has a reddish-brown color. The latter has ectothrix hair infections while *T. simii* shows ecto-endothrix infections. *Trichophyton simii* produces more macroconidia.

5. **Perfect Stage**: *Arthroderma simii* Stockdale, Mackenzie & Austwick, 1965. Cleistothecia globose, pale buff, 200-750 μ in diam. Peridial hyphae hyaline, pale buff, septate, verruculose walls. Some peridial hyphae have spirals, loosely or tightly coiled. Asci sub-globose, evanescent, 5-7.7 μ in diameter, with 8 hyaline, smooth-walled, lenticular ascospores 2.9-3.3 by 1.7-2.1 μ, yellow in mass. Heterothallic.

3. Endothrix Hair Invasion

A. *Trichophyton tonsurans* Malmsten, 1945

  1. **Occurrence**:

    (a) <u>Man</u>: This species usually causes tinea capitis with a black dot appearance from burst and crumbled hair shafts on the scalp due to abundant sporulation inside the hair. Occasionally tinea corporis, tinea pedis, or tinea unguium may occur. Worldwide.

    (b) <u>Animals</u>: Rare, but cases reported in a horse and a dog.

  2. **Colonies** develop fairly slowly on Sabouraud agar, forming raised or sunken centers, and a folded surface with yellowish color in the depressions. The surface of the colony is velvety to powdery with a variation in color from creamy-white, yellow, rose to brown (see Plate IX). Compare with other species.

  3. **Microscopically**, numerous clavate microconidia are attached along the sides of the hyphae or on short sterigmata. The thin-walled, club-shaped macroconidia are rare. Numerous chlamydospores and racquet hyphae may be seen.

  4. **Special Comments**: *T. tonsurans* grows better with the addition of thiamine which helps to separate this species from *T. mentagrophytes,* or *T. rubrum.*

B. *Trichophyton schoenleinii* (Lebert) Langeron and Milochevitch, 1930

  1. **Occurrence**:

    (a) <u>Man</u>: Primarily a favus infection of tinea capitis, at times causing tinea corporis, and at times tinea unguium. The hairs typically have degenerate hyphae or air spaces and hyphae present, with cuplike crusts in the hair follicles (scutula). More common in Eurasia and North Africa and less likely to occur in North or South America.

    (b) <u>Animals</u>: Cases have been reported in a dog, cat, hedgehog, mouse, cow, horse, rabbit, and guinea pig.

  2. **Colonies** are very slow-growing, heaped with many irregular folds, waxy smooth, later, or upon subsequent transfers, becoming velvety white. The color varies from yellowish-white to light brown (see Plate IX). This species grows well at room temperature or 37° C without the addition of vitamins to the medium.

  3. **Microscopically**, the characteristic structures are the "favic chandeliers" even though other species in this group may have the same structures. Chlamydospores or hyphal swellings are commonly found, but no macroconidia have been reported.

  Microconidia may be formed in rare cases, especially on rice grains.

  4. **Special Comments**: No special nutrients needed.

Trichophyton sp—colonies
Endothrix type hair invasion (43-47)
Species not invading hair (48)
Saprophytes in soil (49-50)

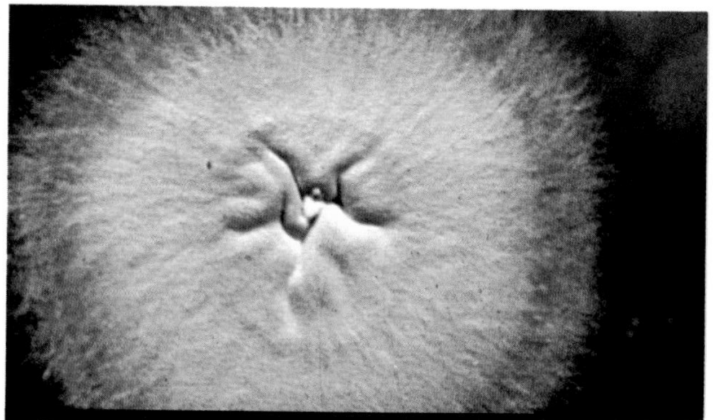

43 T. tonsyrans

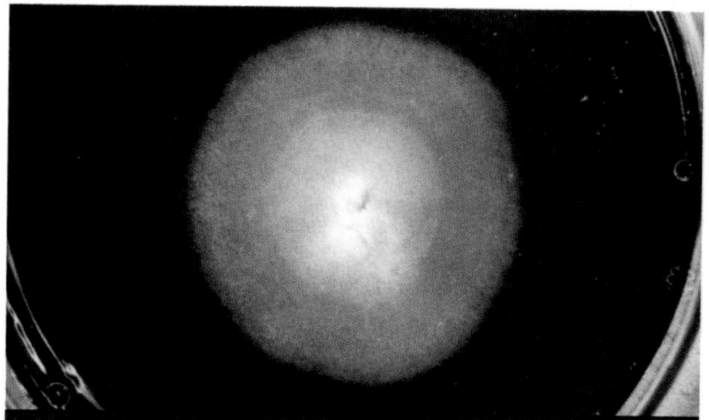

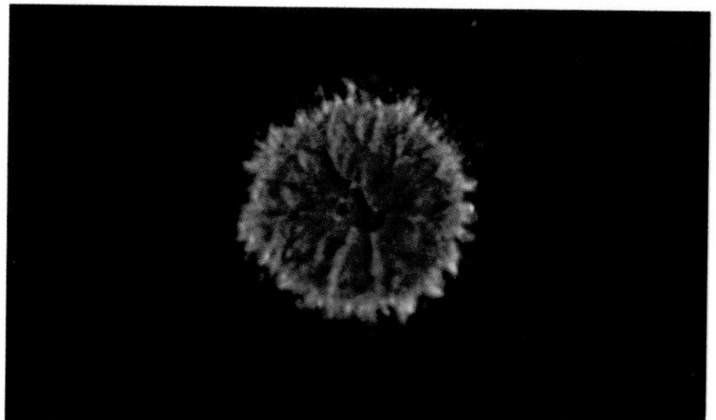

45 T. violaceum

44 T. schoenleinii

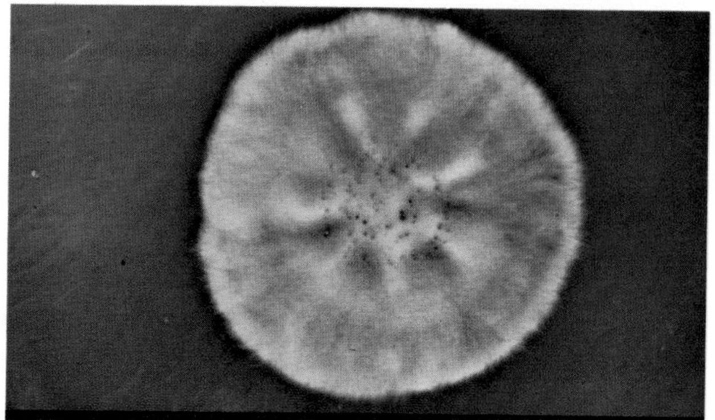

46 T. gourvilii

PLATE IX

C. *Trichophyton violaceum* Sabouraud, apud Bodin, 1902

   1. **Occurrence:**

      (a) <u>Man</u>: Usually a cause of ringworm of the scalp and body (tinea capitis and tinea corporis), at times causes tinea unguium and favuslike symptoms. Present in Europe, North Africa, Russia, Eastern Europe, United States and Brazil.

      (b) <u>Animals</u>: Reported to have infected a calf, dog, cat, horse, mouse, and a pigeon.

   2. **Colonies** are slow-growing (up to 3 or 4 weeks required), forming a heaped, folded, glabrous, waxy surface with a violet color. Later a velvety, aerial mycelium may appear. More vigorous growth occurs with the addition of trypticase and thiamine to Sabouraud glucose agar (see Plate IX). Loss of pigment may occur in variants when transfers are made. Compare colony characteristics with *T. schoenleinii*.

   3. **Microscopically,** chlamydospores and hyphal swellings are the usual mycelial structures seen on Sabouraud agar. Microconidia may occur in small numbers on media enriched with thiamine.

   4. **Special Comments:** All strains are partially dependent on thiamine for growth. Stock cultures should be kept at room temperature in preference to the refrigerator.

D. *Trichophyton gourvilii* Catanei, 1933

   1. **Occurrence:**

      (a) <u>Man</u>: This species is the cause of tinea capitis and tinea corporis in Africa.

      (b) <u>Animals</u>: No known cases.

   2. **Colonies** are somewhat similar to the growth of *T. violaceum* and *T. soudanense*. The surface is folded, heaped, and waxy, later becoming velvety with light lavender to deep garnet-red pigmentation (see Plate IX).

   3. **Microscopically,** microconidia and macroconidia have been reported to occur in some strains.

   4. **Special Comments:** No special nutritional requirements. In contrast, *T. violaceum* needs thiamine and *T. megninii* requires histidine.

F. *Trichophyton soudanense* Joyeux, 1912

   1. **Occurrence:**

      (a) <u>Man</u>: This species primarily causes ringworm of the scalp (tinea capitis) and tinea corporis. Occurs primarily in Africa and occasionally in Brazil, the United States, and Great Britain through immigration of individuals.

      (b) <u>Animals</u>: No known cases.

   2. **Colonies** are slow-growing (5-20 mm in diameter after 10 days), flat, later raised or at times folded in center. Surface is smooth to velvety, lemon yellow to apricot in color (see Plate X). Reverse side of colony is yellow to orange. Variants (pleomorphisms) develop readily.

   3. **Microscopically,** the hyphae separate readily into arthrospores. Numerous or occasional microconidia occur and are ovoid or clavate to pyriform in shape.

   4. **Special Comments:** No special nutrients needed. Stock cultures survive better at room temperature than in the refrigerator.

G. *Trichophyton yaoundei* Cochet and Doby-Dubois, 1957

   1. **Occurrence:**

      (a) <u>Man</u>: This species causes tinea capitis in primarily the Cameroon and Congo areas of Africa.

(b) Animals: No known cases.

2. **Colonies** are slow-growing, very glabrous, raised and folded, and white to cream in color at first, later becoming tan to chocolate brown in a few weeks with some diffusion of the pigment in the medium. There may be some submerged hyphal growth in the medium. Pleomorphic changes or sectors develop.

3. **Microscopically,** numerous chlamydospores form on the irregular hyphae. No macroconidia; microconidia rare.

4. **Special Comments:** No special nutritional requirements. Young colonies may resemble *T. verrucosum* but do not require thiamine for growth.

4. Hairs Not Invaded

A. *Trichophyton concentricum* Blanchard, 1896

1. **Occurrence:**

   (a) Man: This organism is the chief cause of tinea imbricata (tinea corporis with concentric rings of scales on the skin), occurring commonly in South Pacific Islands and also in Guatemala, Southern Mexico, and Central Brazil.

   (b) Animals: No reported cases.

2. **Colonies** are raised, deeply folded, smooth and white at first, becoming cream to amber or brown, and covered with short gray hyphae. The reverse side of the colony is cream to brown in color. Slow-growing, 5-20 mm in diameter after 10 days (see Plate X).

3. **Microscopically,** this organism is similar to strains of *T. schoenleinii*. The swollen hyphae with chlamydospores and aborted hyphal branches are typical. Macroconidia and microconidia are lacking.

4. **Special Comments:** Some strains may grow better with thiamine in the medium (about 50% of the strains).

5. Saprophytes — Found in Soil

A. *Trichophyton georgii* Varsavsky and Ajello, 1964

1. **Occurrence:** The habitat of this nonpathogenic species is soil or hairs of the opossum in the United States.

2. **Colonies** are flat with an umbonate, grayish vinaceous center. The periphery is more granular, pale brownish to vinaceous with a fringed edge. Reverse side of colony is diamine brown, spotted with dark red or vinaceous brown.

3. **Microscopically,** microconidia are abundant, variable in size and shape, elongate-clavate or at times pyriform to subglobose, 1-celled, up to 3-celled on occasions, 4.2-6.4 by 2.0-2.4 μ in size.

4. **Special Comments:** None.

5. **Perfect Stage:** *Arthroderma ciferrii* Varsavsky and Ajello, 1964. Cleistothecia globose, 500-800 μ in diameter with appendages, ochraceous salmon becoming brownish vinaceous with age. Peridium has uncinately branched hyphae with curled ends. Peridial hyphae dumbbell-shaped, asperulate. Appendages two types: smooth-walled, spiralled hyphae, or smooth-walled, tapered hyphae. Asci subglobose, evanescent, with 8 ascospores. Heterothallic.

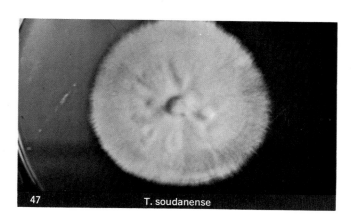

47   T. soudanense

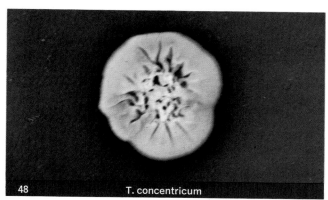

48   T. concentricum

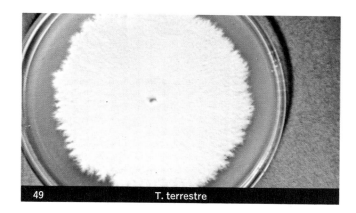

49   T. terrestre

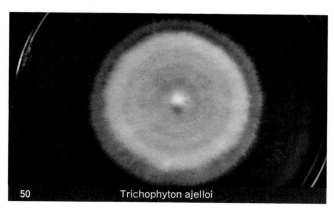

50   Trichophyton ajelloi

PLATE X

B. *Trichophyton terrestre* Durie and Frey, 1957

    1. **Occurrence:** This nonpathogenic species is found in soil throughout the world, and has been isolated from hair of wild rats and horses.

    2. **Colonies** are moderately fast-growing, 15-30 mm in diameter after 10 days, powdery to velvety, resembling *T. mentagrophytes* at times, with a pale lemon yellow to buff surface color. The reverse colony color may be yellow or a reddish color. (See Plate X.)

    3. **Microscopically,** microconidia are clavate with a flat base. Transitional forms from microconidia to several-celled macroconidia may be present. Spiral coils may form.

    4. **Special Comments:** No special nutrients needed.

    5. **Perfect Stage:** *Arthoderma quadrifidum* Dawson and Gentles, 1961. Cleistothecia globose, pale buff, 400-700 μ, average 580 μ in diameter without appendages. The peridial hyphae are pale yellow, hyaline, septate, uncinately branched with cells that are thick-walled, strongly echinulate, dumbbell-shaped when young, maturing into short humerus bonelike forms with condyles on one side. The appendages are septate with spirals of varying length. Subglobose, evanescent asci produce 8 hyaline ascospores that are smooth or finely roughened, lenticular, 1.8-2.7 by 0.9-1.8 μ, and yellow in mass. Heterothallic.

C. *Trichophyton ajelloi* (Vanbreuseghem) Ajello, 1967

    1. **Occurrence:**

        (a) <u>Man</u>: A few cases of tinea corporis have been reported. Considered a rare cause of ringworm.

        (b) <u>Animals</u>: A few rare cases reported in cattle, dogs, a horse, and a squirrel.

    2. **Cultures:** This organism grows readily at room temperature on Sabouraud glucose agar (with the addition of antibiotics if material is contaminated).

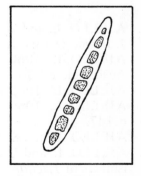

Figure 50

        (a) <u>Colonies</u> grow rapidly, with a flat surface varying from finely powdered to downy, and cream, tan, or orange-tan in color. The reverse side of the colony varies from no pigmentation to reddish or deep bluish-black (see Plate X).

        (b) <u>Microscopically</u>, macroconidia are numerous, cylindrofusiform (cylindric with tapering ends), thick, smooth-walled, with 5 to 12 cells, 20-65 by 5-10 μ in size (Fig. 50). Microconidia usually abundant, pyriform to ovate in shape, sessile.

    3. **Special Comments:** White cottony areas (pleomorphic) develop readily in the colonies.

    4. **Perfect Stage:** *Arthroderma uncinatum* Dawson and Gentles, 1961. Cleisthothecia globose, white to buff, 300-900 μ in size. The peridial hyphae are hyaline, septate, uncinately branched usually away from the main branch of the main hyphae. Cells are thick-walled, echinulate, dumbbell-shaped, and 4-5 μ in diameter. The spirals are smooth-walled, born terminally or laterally on peridial hyphae. The asci are globose, evanescent, 4.9 by 7.2 μ in size, with yellow ascospores.

    5. **Animal Inoculation:** Experimental infections have been obtained in mice, and guinea pigs.

D. Other Saprophytes from Soil

    1. *Trichophyton gloriae* Ajello & Cheng, 1967. This species occurs in soils in California, New Mexico, and Arizona. Macroconidia, 40 μ by 5 μ in size, thin-walled, with 10 septa are

characteristic. The conidia are usually in clusters. The heterothallic perfect stage is *Arthroderma gloriae* Ajello and Cheng 1967. For more details see Ajello and Cheng (1967).

2. *Trichophyton vanbreuseghemii* Rioux, Jarry & Juminer, 1964. This species has been isolated from soil in Tunisia. The macroconidia are thin-walled, 5- to 8-celled, and cylindrical or clavate in shape. The perfect stage is *Arthroderma gertleri* Bohme, 1967. For more information see Rioux, Jarry and Juminer (1964).

Questions:

1. Distinguish *Trichophyton* from *Microsporum* and *Epidermophyton*.

2. How are the *Trichophyton* species separated?

3. Compare the mode of growth of species of *Trichophyton* with *Microsporum* in the hair.

4. Describe the technique for isolation of a dermatophyte, beginning with a lesion on a patient.

5. Compare the appearance of *Malassezia furfur* with *Trichophyton* in skin.

6. Differentiate hair infections with *Corynebacterium tenuis,* black or white piedra, *Microsporum* sp. and *Trichophyton* sp. Can the genus be distinguished in all cases or should cultures be made?

7. After reading some of the current literature on physiological studies of growth of the dermatophytes, compare the effects of various compounds upon the growth of these fungi.

8. Where do the perfect stages of some of the dermatophytes usually occur?

9. Explain why the species in the former genus *Keratinomyces* were transferred to the genus *Trichophyton*.

Selected References

1. AJELLO, L. and M. E. Getz. 1954. Recovery of Dermatophytes from shoes and shower stalls. J. Invest. Derm. 22:17.
2. AJELLO, L. 1960. Geographic distribution and prevalence of the dermatophytes. Ann. N. Y. Acad. Sci. 89:30.
3. AJELLO, L. 1962. Present day concepts of the dermatophytes. Mycopathologia. 17:315.
4. AJELLO, L. 1968. A taxonomic review of the dermatophytes and related species. Sabouraudia. 6:147.
5. AJELLO, L. and S. Y. Cheng. 1967. A new geophilic *Trichophyton.* Mycologia. 59:255.
6. AJELLO, L. and L. K. Georg. 1957. In vitro hair cultures for differentiating between atypical isolates of *Trichophyton mentagrophytes* and *Trichophyton rubrum.* Mycopathologia. 8:3.
7. ANDREWS, G. C., A. N. Domonkos and A. Silva, Jr. 1960. Griseofulvin in dermatomycoses. J. Am. Med. Assoc. 173:1542.
8. BENEKE, E. S. 1953. Detection of mycotic infection in animals. MSC Veterinarian, 13:219.
9. BENHAM, R. W. 1948. Effect of nutrition on growth and morphology of the dermatophytes. I. Development of macroconidia in *Trichophyton rubrum.* Mycologia 40:232.
10. BLANK, F. and H. Prichard. 1962. Epidemic ringworm of the groin. Archs. Derm. 85:410.
11. CALNAN, C. D., N. Djavahiszwili and C. J. Hodgson. 1962. *Trichophyton soudanense* in Britain. Brit. J. Derm. 74:144.
12. CATANEI, A. 1933. Description de *Trichophyton gourvilii* n. sp., agent d'une teigne de l'homme. Bull. Soc. Path. Exot. 25:377.
13. CONNOLE, M. D. 1965. Keratinophillic fungi on cats and dogs. Sabouraudia 4:45.
14. COX, W. A. and J. A. Moore. 1968. Experimental *Trichophyton verrucosum* infections in laboratory animals. J. Comp. Path. 78:35.
15. DAWSON, C. O. 1963. Two new species of *Arthroderma* from the soil from rabbit burrows. Sabouraudia 2:185.

16. DAWSON, C. O. and C. J. Gentles. 1961. The perfect state of *Keratinomyces ajelloi* Vanbreuseghem; *Trichophyton terrestre* Durie and Frey, and *Microsporum nanum* Fuentes. Sabouraudia 1:49.

17. DOSTROVSKY, A., G. Kallner, F. Raubitschek and I. Sagher. 1955. Tinea capitis, an epidemiologic therapeutic and laboratory investigation of 6390 cases. J. Invest. Derm. 24:195.

18. DRUHET, E. 1953. Recherches sur la nutrition des dermatophytes III. L'histidine, facteur de croissance des *Trichophyton* du groupe *rosaceum.* Ann. Inst. Pasteur, 85:791.

19. DVOŘAK, J., Z. Hubálek, and M. Otčenašek. 1968. Survival of dermatophytes in human skin scales. Archs. Derm. 98:540.

20. DVOŘAK, J. and M. Otčenašek. 1969. Mycological Diagnosis of Animal Dermatophytoses. Dr. W. Junk N. V., Publishers, The Hague.

21. DYSON, J. E., Jr. and M. E. Landay. 1963. Differentiation of *Trichophyton rubrum* from *Trichophyton mentagrophytes.* Mycopathologia. 22:6.

22. EMMONS, C. W. 1934. Dermatophytes. Arch. Derm. and Syph. 30:337.

23. ENGLISH, M. P. and M. D. Gibson. 1959. Studies in the epidemiology of the tinea pedis. II. Dermatophytes on the floors of swimming-baths. Brit. Myc. J. 1:1446.

24. ENGLISH, M. P. and P. M. Stockdale. 1968. *Trichophyton proliferans.* sp. nov., a human pathogen. Sabouraudia 6:267.

25. GEORG, L. K. 1956. The role of animals as vectors of human fungus diseases. Trans. N. Y. Acad. Sci. (Ser. II) 18:639.

26. GEORG, L. K. 1956. Studies on *Trichophyton tonsurans.* II. Morphology and laboratory identification. Mycologia 48:354.

27. GEORG, L. K. 1959. Animal ringworm in public health. Diagnosis and nature. U. S. Dept. of Health, Ed. and Welfare, Communicable Disease Center, Atlanta, Ga. 57 pp.

28. GEORG, L. K. 1960. Epidemiology of the dermatophytes: sources of infection, modes of transmission and epidemicity. Ann. N. Y. Acad. Sci. 89:69.

29. GEORG, L. K. and L. B. Camp. 1957. Routine nutritional tests for the identification of dermatophytes. J. Bact. 74:113.

30. GEORG, L. K., P. Doupagne, S. R. Pattyn and H. Neves. 1963. *Trichophyton yaoundei* a dermatophyte indigenous to Africa. J. Invest. Derm. 41:19.

31. GEORG, L. K., W. Kaplan and L. B. Camp. 1957. *Trichophyton equinum* reevaluation of its taxonomic status. J. Invest. Derm. 29:27.

32. GUGNANI, H. C., J. B. Shrivastav, and N. P. Gupta. 1967. Occurrence of *Arthroderma simii* in soil and on hair of small mammals. Sabouraudia 6:77.

33. HALEY, L. D. and M. Stonerod. 1954. The isolation and identification of dermatophytes. Am. J. Med. Tech. 20:27.

34. HAND, E. A. and L. K. Georg. 1955. *Trichophyton tonsurans* ringworm. J. Mich. State. Med. Soc. 54:687.

35. HEJTMANEK, M. and J. Kunert. 1965. A dwarf form of *Keratinomyces ajelloi.* Sabouraudia 4:3.

36. KAPLAN, W., L. K. Georg and L. Ajello. 1958. Recent developments in animal ringworm and their public health implications. Ann. N. Y. Acad. Sci. 70:636.

37. KLEIN, D. T. 1964. Time-temperature interaction in the indication of pleomorphism in *Trichophyton mentagrophytes.* J. Gen. Microbiol. 34:125.

38. LONDERO, A. T. 1962. The geographic distribution and prevalence of dermatophytes in Brazil. Sabouraudia 2:108.

39. MARPLES, M. J. 1962. Some extra-human reservoirs of pathogenic fungi in New Zealand. Trans. Roy. Soc. Trop. Med. and Hyg. 56:91.

40. MIGUENS, M. P. 1968. Un Nuevo dermatofito de origen tropical. *Trichophyton fluviomunense* sp. nov. Sabouraudia 6:312.

41. NEVES, H. 1960. Mycological study of 519 cases of ringworm infections in Portugal. Mycopathologia. 13:121.

42. PHILPOT, C. 1967. The differentiation of *Trichophyton mentagrophytes* from *T. rubrum* by a simple urease test. Sabouraudia 5:189.

43. PIER, A. C. and J. P. Hughes. 1961. *Keratinomyces ajelloi* from skin lesions of a horse. J. Amer. Vet. Med. Assoc. 138:484.

44. RANDHAWA, H. S. and R. S. Snadhu. 1963. On the occurrence of two new species of *Trichophyton* in Indian soils. Mycopathologia. 20:225.

45. RAUBITSCHEK, F. and R. Maoz. 1957. Invasion of nails in vitro by certain dermatophytes. J. Invest. Derm. 28:261.

46. REBELL, G., D. Taplin and H. Blank. 1964. Dermatophytes, Their Recognition and Identification. Dermatology Foundation of Miami. 1020 N.W. 16th St., Miami, Fla. 1st Ed. 58 pp.

47. REES, R. G. 1967. *Arthroderma flavescens* sp. nov. Sabouraudia 6:206.

48. RIOUX, J. A., D. T. Jarry, and B. Juminer. 1964. Un nouveau dermatophyte isolé du sol: *Trichophyton vanbreuseghemii* n. sp. Naturalia Monspel. Ser. Bot. 16:153.

49. RIPPON, J. W. and M. Medenica. 1964. Isolation of *Trichophyton soudanense* in the United States. Sabouraudia 3:301.

50. RIPPON, J. W., A. Eng and F. D. Malkinson. 1968. *Trichophyton simii* infection in the United States. Archs. Derm. 98:615.

51. ROSENTHAL, S. A. and H. Wapnick. 1963. The value of Mackenzie's "Hair brush" technique in the isolation of *T. mentagrophytes* from clinically normal guinea pigs. J. Invest. Derm. 41:5.

52. SABOURAUD, R. 1894. Les Trichophyties humaines. Rueff et Cie., Paris.

53. SCHECHTER, Y., J. W. Landau, N. Dabrowa and V. D. Newcomer. 1968. Disc electrophoretic studies of intraspecific variability of proteins from dermatophytes. Sabouraudia 6:133.

54. SCHMITT, J. A., J. M. Mann and D. Stilwill. 1963. Variation in susceptibility to experimental dermatomycosis in genetic strains of mice. II. Preliminary results with B Alb C and white swiss strains. Mycopathologia. 21:114.

55. SEALE, E. R. and J. B. Richardson. 1960. *Trichophyton tonsurans.* Arch. Derm. 81:87.

56. SILVA, M. 1953. Nutritional studies of the dermatophytes. Factors affecting pigment production. Trans. N. Y. Acad. Sci. 15:106.

57. SMITH, J. M. B. and M. J. Marples. 1963. *Trichophyton mentagrophytes* var. *erinacei.* Sabouraudia. 3:1.

58. STOCKDALE, P. M. 1967. *Nannizzia persicolor.* sp. nov., the perfect state of *Trichophyton persicolor* Sabouraud. Sabouraudia 5:355.

59. STOCKDALE, P. M., D. W. R. Mackenzie and P. K. C. Austwick. 1965. *Arthroderma simii* sp. nov., the perfect state of *Trichophyton simii* (Pinoy) comb. nov. Sabouraudia 4:112.

60. SUDMAN, M. S. and J. A. Schmitt, Jr. 1965. Differentiation of *Trichophyton rubrum* and *Trichophyton mentagrophytes* by pigment production. Appl. Microbiol. 13:290.

61. SWARTZ, H. E. and L. K. Georg. 1955. The nutrition of *Trichophyton tonsurans.* Mycologia 47:475.

62. TAPLIN, D., N. Zaias, G. Rebell and H. Blank. 1969. Isolation and recognition of dermatophytes on a new medium (DTM). Archs. Derm. 99:203.

63. TORRES, G. and L. K. Georg. 1956. A human case of *Trichophyton gallinae* infection. Disease contracted from chickens. Archs. Derm. 74:191.

64. ULBRICH, A. P. and T. H. Bonino. 1960. The incidence of dermatophytosis and potential treatment with griseofulvin. Jour. A. O. A. 59:370.

65. VANBREUSEGHEM, R. 1952. Technique biologique pour l'isolement des dermatophytes du sol. Ann. Soc. belge Med. Trop. 32:173.

66. VARSAVSKY, E. and L. Ajello. 1964. The perfect and imperfect forms of a new keratinophilic fungus *Arthroderma ciferrii* sp. nov., *Trichophyton georgii* sp. nov. Riv. Pat. Veg. 4:351.

67. WEITZMAN, I. and M. Silva-Hutner. 1967. Non-keratinous agar media as substrates for the ascigerous state in certain members of the Gymnoascaceae pathogenic for man and animals. Sabouraudia 5:335.

THE DEEP MYCOSES

The deep mycoses will be considered as two subgroups: the subcutaneous mycoses and the systemic mycoses.

Nearly all of the deep mycoses have been reported in North America, with infections originating from various areas on the continent or from other endemic areas throughout the world. As a result of rapid travel of the population from one continent to another, diseases may appear in an area that would not ordinarily be known to occur.

Some of these deep mycoses are localized or systemic, at times fatal, and are caused by a number of different fungi. These organisms are able to attack a wide range of structures in the body including the internal organs, bone, meninges, subcutaneous tissue, mucous membranes, and skin.

In the study of the deep mycoses in class or in the laboratory, the following general procedure is suggested for each disease:

1. Transfer culture and observe time required for colony development. Compare with older cultures or other strains.

2. Prepare a slide culture wherever possible or a direct mount of the fungus. Retain the mounted slides of the mature fungus sealed with finger nail polish, or other cements, for future study.

3. Inoculate laboratory animals sufficiently in advance for autopsy at the time the disease is being studied in the laboratory. This will establish the pathogenic phase which may be entirely different from the saprophytic phase. These fungi are known as diphasic (or dimorphic).

4. Smears or direct mounts of materials from the lesions of the laboratory animal should be made for study of the tissue phase of the fungus. Histological sections may be made if time permits. Stain the smears or histological sections.

5. Use physiological and immunological studies for each disease where possible.

6. Study prepared slides from cases for tissue phase characteristics.

7. Use audio visual aids that are available for study.

8. Literature references.

SUBCUTANEOUS MYCOSES

The subcutaneous mycoses are infections that usually remain limited to the involvement of the skin and subcutaneous tissues, rarely spreading to the internal organs. The three mycoses of this type are: chromoblastomycosis, mycetoma, and sporotrichosis. The etiological agents of these diseases all have a saprophytic existence in nature. The usual route of infection is through wounds.

MYCETOMA

(Madura Foot, Maduromycosis)

Definition:

Mycetoma is a chronic granulomatous infection usually involving the feet (Plate XI) and occasionally the hands or other areas of the body. The disease is characterized by enlargement, deformity, sinus drainage, and bone destruction. The pus usually contains white, light yellow, red, or black granules.

Etiological Agents:

Various saprophytic fungi have been isolated as causative agents in mycetoma. There are two forms of mycetomas or tumorlike infections: (1) mycotic mycetoma caused by species of the higher fungi, and (2) actinomycotic mycetoma caused by members of the actinomycete group. The more important isolates causing mycotic mycetoma are: *Allescheria boydii* Shear, 1921 (imperfect stage: *Monosporium apiospermum* Saccardo, 1911); *Cephalosporium falciforme* Carrión, 1951; *Madurella mycetomi* (Laveran) Brumpt, 1905; *M. grisea* Mackinnon, Ferrada and Montemayer, 1949, and *Phialophora jeanselmei* (Langeron) Emmons, 1945.

The most common causes of actinomycotic mycetoma are: *Nocardia brasiliensis* (Lindenberg) Castellani and Chalmers, 1913; *Streptomyces madurae* (Vincent) Mackinnon and Artagaveitia-Allende, 1956; *S. somaliensis* (Brumpt) Mackinnon and Artagaveitia-Allende, 1956; and *S. pelletierii* (Laveran) Mackinnon and Artagaveitia-Allende, 1956. A discussion of these organisms will be taken up under nocardiosis. *Nocardia asteroides* (Eppinger) Blanchard, 1896 may be reported in mycetomas. The causative agent may be reported as *N. caviae,* a closely related species. (Note: *Streptomyces madurae* should be *Nocardia madurae* on basis of cell wall type.)

Occurrence:

Most of the saprophytic fungi that have been reported in mycetomas have been found in soil and on plants.

1. **Man:** The disease is more common in the tropical and subtropical regions where shoes are not as frequently worn. Mycetoma has been reported in Africa, India, Europe, South America, Mexico, and North America, as well as other parts of the world on occasions. In the United States *Allescheria boydii* is the most likely etiological agent.

2. **Animals:** Twelve reported cases, including dog, cat, and horse.

Laboratory Procedures

1. **Source of Infected Material:** Pus should be taken from draining fistulas, or in nondrainage areas pus may be aspirated by a sterile needle and syringe for laboratory studies. Pus, currettings, or biopsy tissues should be collected in sterile shallow bottles or Petri dishes. Use sterile gauze compresses to collect granules.

2. **Examination of Infected Materials**: Gross examination of the pus, currettings, or biopsy material should be made for the presence of small, oval, irregularly formed granules which are 0.5 to 2 mm in diameter and white, yellow, red, or black in color.

a. Place the granules in water or 10% potassium hydroxide and examine microscopically.

b. <u>Microscopically</u>, the granules produced by higher fungi often contain pigmented hyphae 2-4 μ in diameter with many swellings or chlamydospores throughout the structure including the periphery. Distinguish between granules developed by actinomycetes and higher fungi, noting the difference in width of the hyphae (about 1 μ in diameter). This is important and should be reported immediately to aid in specific treatment as actinomycotic mycetomas can be treated, while mycotic mycetomas are difficult to treat (see Plate XII).

3. **Cultures**: Colonies of the various fungi develop readily on Sabouraud glucose agar at room temperature. The addition of antibacterial antibiotics is desirable but not cycloheximide, as some etiological agents of mycetomas are sensitive to the latter. Aspirated material may be placed directly on the medium while granules from draining fistulas should be washed in sterile saline to reduce contamination and put on the medium containing antibiotics. Cultures should be incubated at both room temperature and 37° C. Morphological and physiological characteristics are used to identify the etiological agents.

a. <u>Special media for physiological tests</u>:

<u>Gelatin medium for liquefaction test</u> (indicates proteolytic activity).

Heart infusion broth	25 gm
Gelatin	120 gm
Distilled water	1000 ml

Dispense 5 ml per tube after adjusting pH to 7.2 to 7.4 and sterilize.

b. <u>Starch medium for hydrolysis test</u> (indicates amylolytic activity).

Peptone	5 gm
Beef extract	3 gm
Agar	15 gm
Distilled water	1000 ml

10 gm potato starch suspended in 40 ml cold distilled water.

Heat above mixture to dissolve agar, add cold starch solution, and autoclave. After fungus growth occurs on plate, flood with 95% alcohol. A clear zone indicates the area of hydrolysis if present.

4. **Etiological Agents**:

a. *Allescheria boydii* Schear, 1921 (white grains).

<u>Colonies</u> develop rapidly with cottony white, aerial mycelium from cream-colored granules. Older colonies turn gray with a gray to black pigment on the reverse side (see Plate XII, imperfect stage name: *Monosporium apiospermum).*

<u>Microscopically</u>, a slide mount from the colony or a slide culture should show moderately. large, septate hyphae with long or short conidiophores, each terminated by a single oval to pyriform conidium, 5-7 by 8-10 μ in size. Coremia (clusters of conidiophores) may be seen with conidia at the ends of the conidiophores (see Plate XII).

Slide mounts from strains of *A. boydii* which produce the ascigerous stage will show brown cleistothecia, 50-200 μ in diameter. When crushed, evanescent subglobose asci should be seen with 8 elliptical, light-brown colored ascospores, 4.5-5 by 5.7-7 μ in size.

<u>Proteolytic Activity</u>: +

<u>Amylolytic Activity</u>: +

   b. *Cephalosporium falciforme* Carrion, 1951 (white grains).

   Colonies rather slow-growing, cottony or tufted, lavender, buff or pinkish. Reverse currant red in color, occasionally producing a soluble pigment.

   Microscopically, hyphae are colorless, 3-4 μ in diameter. Conidia are sickle-shaped, borne in clusters at the tips of simple conidiophores.

   Proteolytic Activity: Slight.

   Amylolytic Activity: 0.

   c. *Madurella mycetomi* (Laveran) Brumpt, 1905 (brown grains).

   Colonies slow-growing, cottony to membranous, flat or folded, white, ochraceous, or yellow-brown. Colonies grow better at 37° C.

   Microscopically, hyphae are 1-6 μ in diameter with many chlamydospores. Flask-shaped phialide may be produced in some strains. Black sclerotia up to 750 μ in diameter may form on media without sugar.

   Proteolytic Activity: Slight.

   Amylolytic Activity: +

   Carbon Assimilation: Glucose +; galactose +; lactose +; maltose +; sucrose 0.

   d. *Madurella grisea* Mackinnon, Ferrada and Montemayer, 1949 (black grains).

   Colonies slow-growing, velvety tan or gray aerial mycelium over a cerebriform center and radially folded colony. Older colonies may become red to brown in color.

   Microscopically, hyphae may be thin, branched, septate, 1-3 μ in diameter or larger moniliform, 3-5 μ in diameter with budding cells. Both types of hyphae are brownish to black in color. No conidia or sclerotia present.

   Proteolytic Activity: Slight.

   Amylolytic Activity: +

   Carbon Assimilation: Glucose +; galactose +; lactose 0; maltose +; sucrose +. See Cazin (1964) for discussion of lactose reaction. He reported lactose was assimilated or is +.

   e. *Phialophora jeanselmei* (Langeron) Emmons, 1945 (black grains).

   Colonies slow-growing, brown-black, smooth, skinlike and moist on the surface at first, later covered with velvety aerial hyphae. Reverse side of colony black (Plate XII).

   Microscopically, hyphae are at first long rows or chains of budding cells sometimes described as toruloidlike, later developing regular hyphae. *Aureobasidium*-like spore formation may be present at first. Conidia are produced in cuplike or tubelike phialides on the regular hyphae.

   Proteolytic Activity: 0.

   Amylolytic Activity: 0.

   Carbon Assimilation: Glucose +; galactose +; lactose 0; maltose +; sucrose +.

5. **Pathological Studies:** Although the granules may be seen readily in sections stained with hematoxylin and eosin, they should also be Gram-stained to aid in differentiation of bacterial masses and fungus granules. The latter stain also aids in distinguishing the mycelium of *Nocardia* in granules in case this is the causative organism. The hyphae and chlamydospores in the granules developed from higher fungi may be illustrated very well if the pigments are not too dark by the periodic acid-Schiff stain.

6. **Animal Inoculations:** Most laboratory animals are not suitable for injection with the higher fungi that cause mycetoma. Hamsters have been shown to develop sclerotic, granulomatous nodules after intraperitoneal or subcutaneous injections of conidial suspensions of *A. boydii.*

Organisms of the Deep or Systemic Mycoses

ORGANISMS IN CULTURE

ORGANISM IN TISSUE

COLONY

91 Allescheria boydii

92 Hyphae and conidia

93 Granule from mycetoma pedis

94 Phialophora jeanselmei

95 Cephalosporium-conidiophores conidia

96 Cephalosporium sp. colony

Plate XII

Questions:

1. How are the granules which have developed from infection with higher fungi distinguished from those developed by the Actinomycetes?

2. Explain the origin of the name maduromycosis and mycetoma.

Selected References

1. AJELLO, L. 1952. The isolation of *Allescheria boydii* Shear, an etiologic agent of mycetomas, from soil. Am. J. Trop. Med. and Hyg. 1:227.
2. ARONSON, S. M., Benham, R. and A. Wolf. 1953. Maduromycosis of the central nervous system. J. Neuropath. 12:158.
3. BORELLI, D. 1962. *Madurella mycetomi y Madurella grisea.* Arch. Venez. Med. Trop. Parasit. Med. 4:195.
4. BERGERON, J. R., J. F. Mullins, and L. Ajello. 1969. Mycetoma caused by *Nocardia pelletieri* in the United States. Archs. Derm. 99:564.
5. BRODEY, R. S., H. F. Schryver, H. F. Deubler, M. Josephine, W. Kaplan, and L. Ajello. 1967. Mycetoma in a dog. J. Am. Vet. Med. Assoc. 151:442.
6. CARRION, A. L. 1951. *Cephalosporium falciforme* n. sp., a new etiologic agent of maduromycosis. Mycologia 43:522.
7. CAZIN, J. and D. W. Decker. 1964. Carbohydrate nutrition and sporulation of *Allescheria boydii.* J. Bact. 88:1624.
8. COCKSHOTT, W. P. and A. M. Rankin. 1960. Medical treatment of mycetoma. Lancet 2:1112.
9. CREITZ, J. and H. W. Harris. 1955. Isolation of *Allescheria boydii* from sputum. Am. Rev. Tuberc. 71:126.
10. EMMONS, C. W. 1944. *Allescheria boydii* and *Monosporium apiospermum.* Mycologia 36:188.
11. EMMONS, C. W. 1945. *Phialophora jeanselmei* comb. n. from mycetoma of the hand. Arch. Path. 39:364.
12. KLOKKE, A. H., G. Swamidasan, R. Anguli, and A. Verghese. 1968. The causal agents of mycetoma in South India. Trans. R. Soc. Trop. Med. Hyg. 62:509.
13. MACKINNON, J. 1962. Mycetomas as opportunistic wound infections. Lab. Invest. 11:1124.
14. MONTES, L. F., R. G. Freeman, and W. McClarin. 1969. Maduromycosis due to *Madurella grisea.* Report of the fifth North American case. Archs. Derm. 99:74.
15. NEUHAUSER, I. 1955. Black grain maduromycosis caused by *Madurella grisea.* Archs. Derm. 72:550.
16. NIELSON, H. S. 1967. Effects of amphotericin B in vitro on perfect and imperfect strains of *Allescheria boydii.* Appl. Microbiol. 15:86.
17. NIELSEN, H. S., N. F. Conant, T. Weinberg, and J. F. Reback. 1968. Report of a mycetoma due to *Phialophora jeanselmei* and undescribed characteristics of the fungus. Sabouraudia 6:330.
18. RIPPON, J. W. and G. L. Peck, 1967. Experimental infection with *Streptomyces madurae* as a function of collagenase. J. Invest. Derm. 49:371.
19. ZAIAS, N. D. Taplin, and G. Rebell. 1969. Mycetoma. Archs. Derm. 99:215.

CHROMOBLASTOMYCOSIS

(Chromomycosis)

Definition:

Chromoblastomycosis is a chronic skin disease characterized by the development of warty or tumorlike lesions which may ulcerate. These cauliflowerlike growths are usually developed on the lower extremities and occasionally on the hands, face, ear, neck, chest, shoulders, and buttocks (see Plate XI).

The disease is caused by dematiaceous fungi. The organism in contaminated soil is usually introduced into the tissue or skin by a splinter or abrasion of the skin.

Etiological Agents:

A variety of dematiaceous fungi may be the cause of the disease. There are at least 5 organisms: (a) *Fonsecaea pedrosoi* (Brumpt, 1922) Negroni, 1936 (synonymy: *Phialophora pedrosoi* Emmons in Binford, et al., 1944; *Hormodendrum pedrosoi* Brumpt, 1922); (b) *Fonsecaea compactum* Carrión, 1940 (*Phialophora compactum* Emmons in Binford et al., 1944; *Hormodendrum compactum* Carrión, 1935); (c) *Phialophora verrucosa* Thaxter in Medlar, 1915 (Synonymy: *Fonsecaea pedrosoi* var. *phialophorica* Carrión, 1940); (d) *Cladosporium carrionii* Trejos, 1954 (Synonymy: *Fonsecaea pedrosoi* var. *cladosporium* Simson, 1946); (e) *Phialophora dermatitidus* (Kano, 1937) Emmons 1963 (synonymy: *Fonsecaea dermatitidis* Carrión, 1950; *Hormodendrum dermatitidis* Conant, 1935; *Hormiscium dermatitidis* Kano, 1937).

For a more detailed discussion of the variations in ideas on the taxonomic position and nomenclature of these organisms, reference should be made to the publications of Emmons (1963), Binford et al., (1944), and Carrión and Silva (1947).

Occurrence:

1. **Man:** Worldwide in distribution, including reports of cases in North, Central, and South America, Dominican Republic, Cuba, Costa Rica, Puerto Rico, Jamaica, Africa, Australia, Russia, and occasionally in other parts of the world.

2. **Animals:** A case was reported to have occurred in a horse in Turkey.

Laboratory Procedures

1. **Source of Infected Material:** Crusts from warty lesions or exudates may be isolated directly on the proper agar medium or put in a sterile container for subsequent examination.

2. **Examination of Infected Material:**

   a. Place crusts from the lesions on a slide with 10% potassium hydroxide add a cover glass, and examine. Exudates may be examined directly on a slide with a cover glass or may be placed in lactophenol cotton blue and sealed with nail polish. For more permanent mounts, as suggested by Borelli (1957), thin scales may be placed in a drop of xylene on a slide, Canada balsam or other mounting medium added and a cover glass placed on top.

   b. <u>Microscopically</u>, the organisms are single-celled or clustered, round, thick-walled, with a dark-brown or black pigment, and multiply by cross-wall formation (splitting), not budding. The size varies from 6 to 12 μ in diameter. Note the thick-walled structure in Plate XIII. All the organisms causing chromoblastomycosis have the same appearance in tissue.

3. **Cultures:** All of the organisms can be isolated on Sabouraud glucose agar at room temperature. Infected material should be retained in culture for at least three weeks before the plates are considered negative. Cycloheximide or chloramphenicol may be added for the selective isolation of these organisms. Identification of the cultures is based on their morphological and physiological characteristics.

   a. *Fonsecaea pedrosoi* (Brumpt, 1922) Negroni, 1936 (Plate XIII).

      <u>Colonies</u> are slow-growing, dark-green to brown or black on Sabouraud glucose agar, with a feltlike aerial mycelium (see Plate XIII). Strains of the organism show variation in rate of growth and colony characteristics.

Organisms of the Deep or Systemic Mycoses

COLONY

ORGANISMS IN CULTURE

ORGANISM IN TISSUE

97 Phialophora verrucosa

98 Conidiophores with microconidia

99 Chromoblastomycosis-dividing cells

100 Fonsecaea pedrosoi

101 Conidiophore

102 Fonsecaea compactum colony

PLATE XIII

Microscopically, three different methods of conidial formation may be seen, depending upon the strain. Look for these three types in a slide culture or slide mount under the microscope.

(1) The *Cladosporium* type is characterized by branching conidiophores with chains of conidia borne terminally. The single-celled conidia are 3 to 6 μ in length and 1.5 to 3 μ in diameter. Separate conidia are brown to green in color, with projections on the ends which represent the previous junction of one conidium with another (Plate XIII). The *Cladosporium* type conidial formation usually predominates for *P. pedrosoi*.

(2) The *Acrotheca* type has conidia formed along the sides of swollen, knotted, club-shaped conidiophores that developed terminally or laterally on the hyphae.

(3) The *Phialophora* type has conidia developed endogenously or cut off from the base of a terminal caplike structure on a flask-shaped conidiophore (Plate XIII).

Biochemical reactions: Does not hydrolyze starch, coagulate milk, or liquefy gelatin.

b. *Fonsecaea compactum* Carrion, 1940. (Plate XIII).

Colonies of this fungus grow extremely slow on Sabouraud glucose agar forming a heaped, brittle colony, dark-green to black in color with short aerial mycelium. After a month, tufts of brown-colored mycelium develop in the center of the colony containing conidiophores (see Plate XIII). *Phialophora* type conidiophores may form on corn meal agar cultures.

Microscopically, a slide mount from the mycelial tufts in the center of the colony or a slide culture should show terminal and lateral conidiophores with chains of nearly spherical conidia formed close together as compact heads (see Plate XIII). The conidia are 1. 5-2 by 2-3 μ in size (Plate XIII). Slide mounts from cornmeal agar cultures may show the *Phialophora* type conidiophores.

Biochemical reactions: Does not hydrolyze starch, coagulate milk, or liquefy gelatin.

c. *Phialophora verrucosa* Thaxter in Medlar, 1915 (Plate XIII).

Colonies develop slowly and become greenish-brown to black in color with olive to gray colored mycelium closely matted to the surface (see Plate XIII).

Microscopically, conidia are produced in clusters from cups at the tips of the conidiophores while a direct mount on a slide will frequently disperse the clusters of conidia, and consequently the conidia may appear separate. The conidiophores are about 3-4 μ wide and 4-7 μ in length, while the conidia are thin-walled oval cells about 1.5 by 4 μ in size. Higher magnifications should be used to observe these structures (see Plate XIII).

Biochemical reactions: Does not hydrolyze starch, coagulate milk, or liquefy gelatin.

d. *Cladosporium carrionii* Trejos 1954.

Colonies of this organism grow slowly, reaching a diameter of 2 to 4 cm in about one month. The colonies are flat with a slight raise in the center covered with short mycelium on the surface, and a velvety gray-green to brown color.

Microscopically, the *Cladosporium* type lateral and terminal conidiophores are seen with long, branched chains of smooth-walled conidia that separate readily on a slide mount. The *Acrotheca* and *Phialophora* types of conidiophores are lacking. This fungus appears similar to the saprophytic *Cladosporium* species.

Biochemical reactions: Does not hydrolyze starch, coagulate milk, or liquefy gelatin.

e. *Phialophora dermatitidis* (Kano, 1937) Emmons, 1963.

Colonies are of two types. The young colonies are black, soft, moist, shiny and yeastlike. After about a month, the periphery of the colony develops a mycelial growth that changes the colony to a more filamentous type. Sectors may appear.

Microscopically, notice the oval to round budding yeastlike cells in the slide mounts from young colonies, while older colonies have slender hyphae with slight projections along the sides producing budding cells as in *Aureobasidium*. The *Cladosporium* type conidiophore with conidia separating into clusters is rare on hyphal branches. Rarely will a terminal cup of the *Phialophora* type be present.

Biochemical reactions: Does not hydrolyze starch, coagulate milk, or liquefy gelatin.

f. *Cladosporium* species (formerly *Hormodendrum)*.

Colonies of the saprophytic forms vary from flat to irregularly heaped and folded, moderately fast-growing, surface velvety, olive-green to grayish-green with a greenish-black undersurface.

Microscopically, the hyphae are brown to olive in color, with branched conidiophores of varied lengths containing branching chains of conidia. New conidia form by budding at the tips of the chains, but later may form two-celled conidia.

Biochemical reactions: Hydrolyzes starch, coagulates milk, and liquefies gelatin.

4. **Animal Inoculation**: Intraperitoneal injection of saline suspensions of the fungi into rats or mice is successful as these animals are more susceptible. Lesions have been developed in rabbits, guinea pigs, dogs, and monkeys. Cultures rather than animal inoculation are usually made in the laboratory for an accurate diagnosis of the etiological agent.

a. *Procedure:*

(1) Heavy suspensions of spores and mycelium from cultures 1 to 1½ months old, or ground surface growth from liquid Sabouraud glucose medium 96 hours after inoculation, should be placed in physiological saline solution, and ½ ml injected into mice or rats intraperitoneally or intratesticularly.

(2) Mice or rats inoculated intraperitoneally should develop granulomas in the abdominal cavity after a few weeks. Look for these near the site of the injection. If rats are inoculated intratesticularly check for inflammatory orchitis.

(3) Look for the characteristic cells of the organisms on smears or in frozen stained sections of material from biopsy or autopsy of the animal.

Questions:

1. Distinguish between the different fungi causing chromoblastomycosis in the form of a table or chart.

2. What is the meaning of the term chromoblastomycosis? Why is this word misleading for this disease?

3. Under what family and order would these organisms be placed in the deuteromycetes?

Selected References

1. AJELLO, L. and L. Runyon. 1953. Abortive "perithecial" production by *Phialophora verrucosa*. Mycologia 45:947.
2. BARWASSER, N. C. 1953. Chromoblastomycosis, thirteenth reported case in the United States. J. Am. Med. Assoc. 153:556.
3. BEERMAN, H. and L. M. Solomon. 1963. Amphotericin B and electrodesiccation for chromoblastomycosis. Arch. Derm. 87:492.
4. BERGER, L., M. Beaudry and E. Gaumond. 1945. Chromoblastomycosis due to a new species of fungus. Canad. Med. Assoc. J. 53:138.

5. BINFORD, C. H., G. Hess and C. W. Emmons. 1944. Chromoblastomycosis. Report of a case from continental United States and discussion of the classification of the causative fungus. Arch. Derm. and Syph. 49:398.

6. CAMPINS, H. and M. Scharvj. 1953. Chromoblastomicosis. Comentarios sobre 34 casos, con estudio clínico, histólogico y micológico. Gac. méd. Carácas 61:127.

7. CARRIÓN, A. L. 1950. Yeastlike dematiaceous fungi infecting the human skin: Special reference to the so-called *Hormiscium dermatitidis.* Arch. Derm. and Syph. 61:996.

8. CARRIÓN, A. L. 1950. Chromoblastomycosis. Ann. N. Y. Acad. Sci. 50:1255.

9. CARRIÓN, A. L. and M. Silva. 1947. Chromoblastomycosis and its etiologic fungi *in* Biology of Pathogenic Fungi. W. J. Nickerson, Editor, Chronica Botanica Co., Waltham, Mass.

10. CONANT, N. F. and D. S. Martin. 1937. The morphologic and seroligic relationships of the various fungi causing dermatitis verrucosa (chromoblastomycosis). Am. J. Trop. Med. 17:553.

11. COSTELLO, M. J., C. P. De Feo and M. L. Littman. 1959. Chromoblastomycosis treated with local infiltration of Amphotericin B. solution. Arch. Derm. 79:184.

12. EMMONS, C. W. and A. L. Carrión. 1936. The Phialophora type of sporulation in *Hormodendrum pedrosoi* and *Hormodendrum compactum.* Puerto Rico J. Pub. Hlth. Trop. Med. 11:703.

13. FRENCH, A. J. and S. R. Russlee. 1953. Chromoblastomycosis. Report of first case recognized in Michigan, apparently contacted in South Carolina. Arch. Derm. Syph. 67:127.

14. FUENTES, C. A. and Z. E. Bosch. 1960. Biochemical differentiation of the etiological agents of chromoblastomycosis from non-pathogenic *Cladosporium* species. J. Inv. Derm. 36:419.

15. FUKUSHIRO, R., S. Kagawa, S. Nishiyama et H. Takahashi. 1957. Un cas de chromoblastomycose cutanée avec métastase cérébrale mortelle. Presse Med. 65:2142.

16. GORDON, M. A. and Y. Al-Doory. 1965. Application of fluorescent-antibody procedures to the study of pathogenic dematiaceous fungi. Serological relationships of the genus *Fonsecaea.* J. Bact. 89:551.

17. HUGHES, W. B. 1967. Chromoblastomycosis: successful treatment with topical amphotericin B. J. Pediat. 71:351.

18. IWATA, K. and T. Wada. 1957. Mycological studies on the strains isolated from a case of chromoblastomycosis with a metastasis in central nervous system. Jap. J. Microbiol. 1:355.

19. KARRER, H. and N. F. Conant. 1953. A cleistotheciumlike structure found in *Hormodendrum pedrosoi.* Mycologia 45:693.

20. LANE, C. G. 1915. Cutaneous disease caused by new fungus (*Phialophora verrucosa*). J. Cutan. Dis. 33:840.

21. Mc GILL, H. C. and J. W. Brueck. 1956. Brain abscess due to *Hormodendrum* species. Arch. Path. 62:303.

22. MEDLAR, E. M. 1915. A cutaneous infection caused by a new fungus *Phialophora verrucosa* with a study of the fungus. J. Med. Res. 32:507.

23. NIELSEN, H. S., Jr., and N. F. Conant. 1968. A new human pathogenic *Phialophora.* Sabouraudia 6:228.

24. SILVA, M. 1958. The saprophytic phase of the fungi of chromoblastomycosis: Effect of nutrients and temperature upon growth and morphology. Trans. N. Y. Acad. Sci. 21:46.

25. SILVA, M. 1960. Growth characteristics of the fungi of chromoblastomycosis. Ann. N. Y. Acad. Sci. 89:17.

26. SIMPSON, J. F. 1966. A case of chromoblastomycosis in a horse. Vet. Med. Small Anim. Clin. 61:1207.

27. TREJOS, A. 1955. *Cladosporium Carrionii* n. sp. and the problem of Cladosporia isolated from chromoblastomycosis. Rev. Biol. Trop. 2:75.

28. WILSON, J. W. 1961. Therapy of systemic fungous infections in 1961. Arch. Int. Med. 108:292.

SPOROTRICHOSIS

Definition:

Sporotrichosis is a chronic infection characterized by nodular lesions and ulcers in the lymph nodes, skin, or subcutaneous tissues, and occasionally in internal organs. The disseminated form may involve the skeletal and visceral areas. The localized lesions are usually found on the hands, arms, or legs (Plate XI).

Etiological Agent:

Sporothrix schenckii Hektoen and Perkins, 1900 (Synonymy: *Sporotrichum schenckii* Matruchot, 1910).

Occurrence:

The fungus has been isolated from soil, wood, and vegetation. The organisms may be injected through wounds from infected splinters or thorns.

1. **Man:** Sporotrichosis is worldwide in distribution, being less frequent in France after 1920 than prior to this date. It periodically occurs in South, Central, and North America. Epidemics have occurred in gold mines of South Africa.

2. **Animals:** Infections have been reported in horses, mules, donkeys, cattle, dogs, fowl, camels, rats, and mice.

Laboratory Procedures

1. **Source of Infected Material:** Pus should be aspirated from unruptured nodules; swabs, scrapings, or biopsies of ulcerated lesions should be collected in a sterile container for laboratory study.

2. **Examination of Infected Materials:**

   a. Pus or other infected material may be put on a slide smeared and stained for examination of the "cigar bodies." However, the fungus is rarely seen in fresh preparations. The use of PAS or methenamine silver stains and the fluorescent antibody techniques may be of value as the presence of only a few organisms will stand out in sharp contrast.

3. **Cultures:** Pus from open lesions or from unopened nodules should be streaked or placed on Sabouraud glucose agar containing cycloheximide and chloramphenicol. Colonies, cream to white in color, will appear in 3 to 5 days and later develop a brown-black pigment.

   a. Colonies at Room Temperature: White at first; leathery, wrinkled, and smooth as the colonies become older. Strains vary from cream to black in color. (see Plate XIV.)

   Colonies at 37° C. This organism can be converted into the tissue phase by growth on media rich in protein and vitamins at 37° C. The use of brain-heart infusion agar with or without blood, or Francis' glucose cystine blood agar at 37° C., are satisfactory media for conversion to the yeast or tissue phase after one or two serial transfers. The medium should be kept moist during the conversion. The colonies appear soft, white to cream in color with an irregular surface somewhat resembling yeast colonies.

   b. Microscopically, a slide mount of a portion of a colony grown at 37° C. should show round, oval, and fusiform budding cells, commonly called "cigar-bodies". (Plate XIV). These are similar to those seen in stained smears from infected laboratory animals. These cells are Gram-positive when stained. Prepare a Gram-stained slide of the yeast phase.

Organisms of the Deep or Systemic Mycoses

ORGANISM IN TISSUE

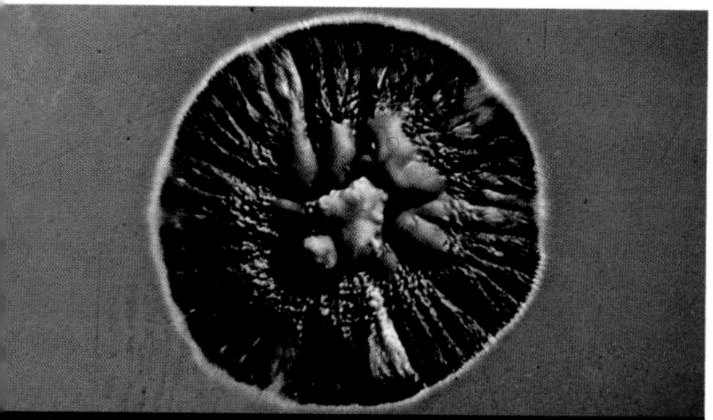

Organism in tissue

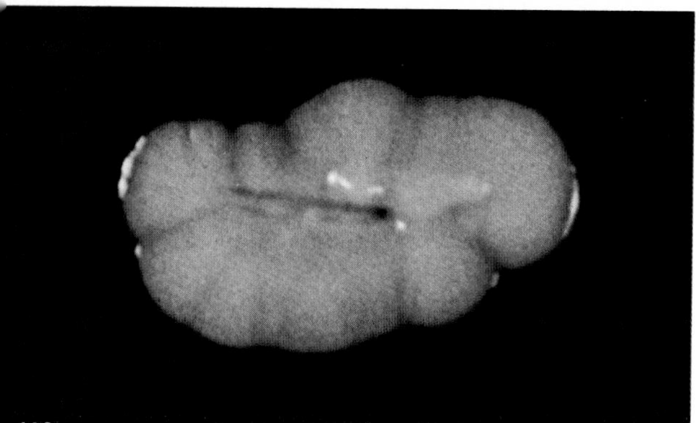

105

Smear—mouse testes

108

ORGANISMS IN CULTURE

Mycelia and conidia

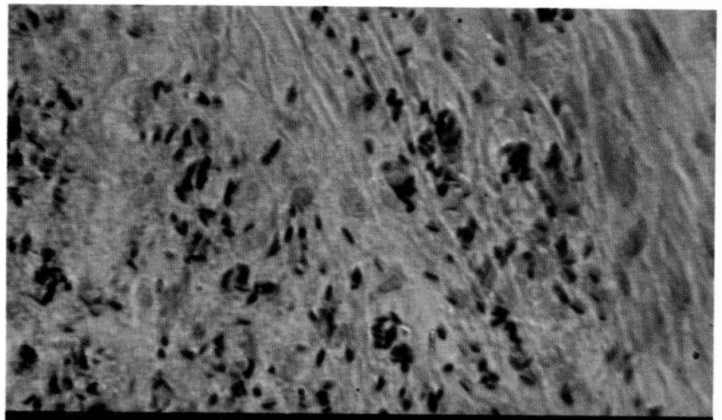

104

Budding cells

107

COLONY

Sporotrichum schenckii

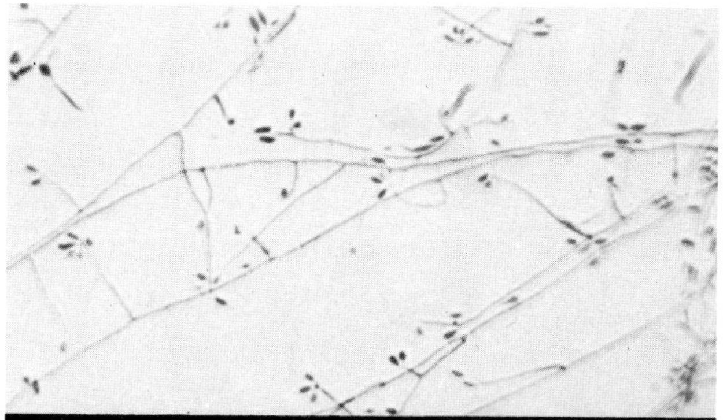

103

S. schenckii colony 37° C

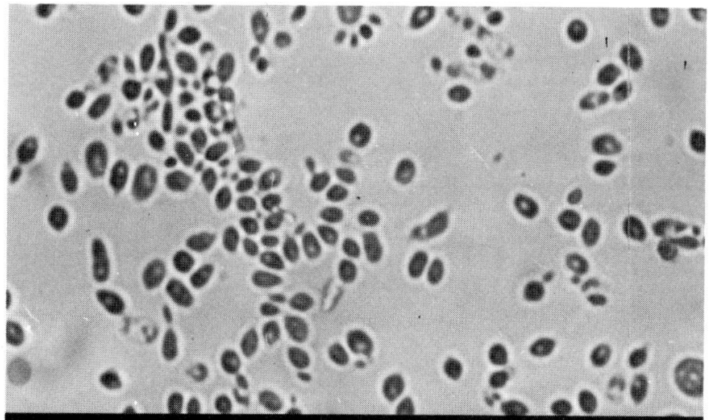

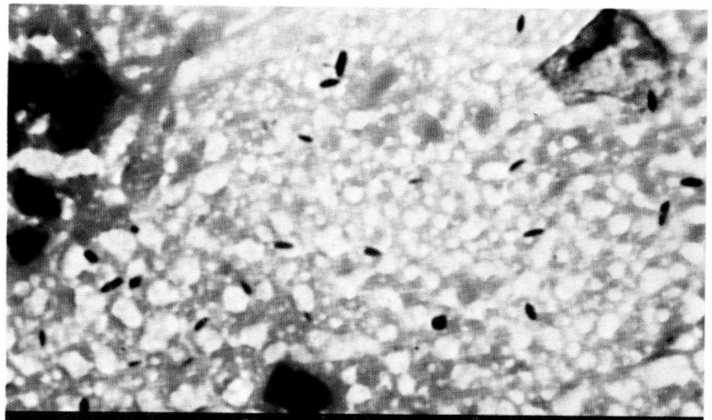

106

PLATE XIV

Microscopically, slide cultures or mounts from colonies grown at room temperature show fine branching, septate hyphae (2 μ in diameter) with pyriform to spherical conidia borne at the ends of minute sterigmata on the tips of conidiophores or on the sides of hyphae resulting in a floral-like arrangement. The conida are 2-4 by 2-6 μ in size (Plate XIV). Compare these with the saprophytic fungus, *Cephalosporium* sp.

4. **Special Nutritional Requirements**.

Yeast Phase. Important factors are: Thiamine, biotin (stimulatory), organic nitrogen source (amino acids), CO_2 tension of 5%; and 37° C., for conversion and growth of the yeast phase of *S. schenckii*.

Mycelial phase. Thiamine is required, organic nitrogen is stimulatory, while inorganic nitrogen can be utilized in culture media.

5. **Histopathological Studies**: Routine H and E stained sections from human tissue rarely show "cigar bodies." The sections may show a nonspecific, inflammatory process or appear granulomatous with infiltration of lymphocytes, giant cells, fibrosis, or other changes. As previously indicated, the use of PAS or Gomori methenamine silver stain or the FA technique will show the organisms when present both within and outside the leucocytes or giant cells. In addition to "cigar-shaped" bodies, asteroid bodies are occasionally seen in tissue sections.

6. **Immunology**: Agglutinins, precipitins, and complement fixing antibodies can be demonstrated, although routine procedures are not usually done in the laboratory.

The fluorescent antibody technique (Kaplan and Ochoa, 1963) has been used as a fast screening procedure in the serologic diagnosis of sporotrichosis and for the identification of the fungus culture.

Small amount of lesion exudates from suspects are placed on slides in a 1-2 cm area, air-dried, heat-fixed, and covered with fluorescein isothiocyanate-labeled rabbit anti-*S. schenckii* globulins and incubated in a moist chamber at 37° C. for 30 minutes. A replicate smear with normal globulin should be made each time for control. The slide is rinsed in saline 10 minutes and water for 5 minutes, air dried, and a drop of 9:1 glycerol phosphate-buffered saline is put on the slide with a cover glass placed on top. The slide is examined with the fluroescent microscope.

7. **Animal Inoculation**: Rats, mice, male hamsters, cats, dogs, and monkeys are susceptible to the disease. Pus or 0.5 to 1.0 ml saline suspensions of the cells from the yeast phase, or mycelial fragments and conidia from the filamentous cultures, should be inoculated intraperitoneally into white mice or rats. Autopsy should be done after three weeks. Look for peritonitis and granulomas in the mesentery of the infected animal. Male animals should show severe orchitis.

The male mouse or other laboratory animal may be inoculated intratesticularly with 0.2 ml of the fungal suspension to produce orchitis in 2 to 3 weeks.

a. Prepare smears from pus or granular material from the animal and use PAS or Gram stain. The cigar-shaped cells of varied shapes should be evident under the immersion oil lens (Plate XIV). The cells are about 1-2 μ in diameter and 4-5 μ in length while the round forms are 2 or 3 μ in diameter. Look for budding forms.

b. To prove Koch's postulates, try isolation of the infected material in culture at 37° C. and room temperature.

Questions:

1. Where is *Sporothrix* sp. found in nature?

2. Are there any other genera of saprophytic fungi that resemble *Sporothrix?*

Selected References

1. BAKER, R. D. 1947. Experimental sporotrichosis in mice. Am. J. Trop. Med. 27:749.
2. BENHAM, R. W. and B. Kesten. 1932. Sporotrichosis: Its transmission to plants and animals. J. Infect. Dis. 50:437.
3. CAMPBELL, C. C. 1945. Use of Francis' glucose cystine blood in the isolation and cultivation of *Sporotrichum schenckii.* J. Bact. 50:233.
4. DROUHET, E. and F. Mariat. 1952. Étude des facteurs déterminant le développement de la phase levure de *Sporotrichum schenckii.* Ann. Inst. Pasteur 83:506.
5. FETTER, B. F. 1961. Human cutaneous sporotrichosis due to *Sporotrichum schenckii;* technique for demonstration of organisms in tissues. Arch. Path. 71:416.
6. FISHBURN, F. and D. C. Kelley. 1967. Sporotrichosis in a horse. J. Am. Vet. Med. Assoc. 151:45.
7. HEKTOEN, L. and C. F. Perkins. 1900. Refractory subcutaneous abscesses caused by *Sporotrix schenckii,* a new pathogenic fungus. J. Exp. Med. 5:77.
8. KAPLAN, W. and M. S. Ivans. 1960. Fluorescent antibody staining of *Sporotrichum schenckii* in cultures and clinical materials. J. Invest. Derm. 35:151.
9. KAPLAN, W. and A. G. Ochoa. 1963. Application of the fluorescent antibody technique to the rapid diagnosis of sporotrichosis. J. Lab. Clin. Med. 62:835.
10. LURIE, H. I. 1951. *Sporotrichum* species; their nitrogen metabolism. Mycologia 43:117.
11. LURIE, H. I. and W. F. S. Still. 1969. The "capsule" of *Sporotrichum schenckii* and the evolution of the asteroid body. A light and electron microscopic study. Sabouraudia 7:64.
12. MARIAT, F. and E. Drouhet. 1953. Action de la biotine sur la croissance de *Sporotrichum schenckii.* Ann. Inst. Pasteur 84:659.
13. MARIAT, F. and E. Drouhet. 1954. Sporotrichose expérimentale du hamster. Observation de formes astéroides de *Sporotrichum.* Ann. Inst. Pasteur 86:485.
14. NIELSEN, H. S. 1968. Biological properties of skin test antigens of yeast from *Sporotrichum schenckii.* J. Infect. Dis. 118:173.
15. NORDEN, A. 1951. Sporotrichosis. Clinical and laboratory features and a serologic study in experimental animals and humans. Acta Path. Microbiol. Scand., Suppl. 89, 119 pp., 14 Figs., 11 Graphs.
16. POST, G. W., A. Jackson, P. E. Garber and G. E. Veach. 1958. Pulmonary sporotrichosis. Dis. Chest 34:455.
17. REID, J. D. 1952. A modified Sabouraud medium for the cultivation and identification of *Sporotrichum schenckii.* Am. J. Clin. Path. 22:1030.
18. SAUNDERS, L. Z. 1948. Systemic fungus infections in animals: A review. Cornell Vet. 38:213.
19. SCHOEMAKER, E. H., H. D. Bennett, W. S. Fields, F. C. Whitcomb and B. Halpert. 1957. Leptomeningitis due to *Sporotrichum schenckii.* Arch. Path. 64:222.
20. SIMSON, F. W. 1947. *Sporotrichosis Infection on Mines of the Witwatersrand.* A symposium. Transvaal Chamber of Mines, Johannesburg.
21. WALLK, S. and G. Bernstein. 1964. Systemic sporotrichosis with bony involvement. Arch. Derm. 90:355.

THE SYSTEMIC MYCOSES

The systemic mycoses may involve all of the internal organs of the body and in some stages the skin as well. Some of the mycoses involve the bone as well as the subcutaneous tissue. In many cases the systemic mycoses may be asymptomatic and can be recognized only by immunological procedures, while other cases may be mild and self-limited. In the progressive form of the disease the symptoms are pronounced, internal organs may be damaged, and death may occur if the patient does not respond to chemotherapy.

Many of the systemic mycoses appear entirely different in tissue in contrast to the culture phase. These fungi are referred to as "diphasic" organisms. Fungi causing South American blastomycosis, North American blastomycosis, coccidioidomycosis, histoplasmosis, candidiasis, and the previously mentioned sporotrichosis and chromoblastomycosis are typical examples of this phenomenon.

NORTH AMERICAN BLASTOMYCOSIS

(Gilchrist's Disease)

Definition:

This disease is a chronic verrucose, granulomatous, and suppurative mycotic infection that may occur in three clinical forms: cutaneous, pulmonary, and systemic (see Plate XI). Symptoms may be similar to tuberculosis. The fungus involved causes infections, especially in the skin, lungs, and bones. The infections may occur in the pulmonary form or dissemination may occur involving the skin, the osseous system, central nervous system, urogenital system, and other organs. Cutaneous blastomycosis is a rare form of the disease. The infection may involve any organ of the body except the intestinal tract.

Etiological Agent:

Blastomyces dermatitidis Gilchrist and Stokes 1898.

Perfect state: *Ajellomyces dermatitidis* McDonough and Lewis 1968.

Occurrence:

1. **Man:** North American blastomycosis is found chiefly in North America. Reports of cases from other areas of the world in certain instances have not been cultured or correctly diagnosed. A few cases have been reported in Mexico, Central America, northern South America, Tunisia, and recently in Africa (Emmons et al., 1964).

2. **Animals:** A number of cases of blastomycosis in dogs have been reported in North America. Cases in a horse, a mare, and a sea lion have also been reported.

3. **Soil:** The fungus has been recovered from soil samples.

Laboratory Procedures

1. **Source of Infected Material:** *B. dermatitidis* can be most easily isolated from multiple minute abscesses in skin lesions. Scrapings, small pieces of tissue, sputum, or pus from the edge of the skin lesion should be collected. Pus from subcutaneous abscesses should be aspirated with a sterile syringe and needle, and sputum, urine, and spinal fluid should be submitted in suspected systemic cases. In case of bone infection, material should be collected from this area for examination in the laboratory.

2. **Examination of Infected Materials:**

   a. Pus from human cases should be placed as a drop on a slide (being sure to use sterile technique) and pressed down with a cover glass. If there are no budding cells in the pus, ring the cover glass with petrolatum, and in a couple hours single germ tubes form for this genus. If opaque material is present, put 10% potassium hydroxide on a slide with a cover glass. To keep infected pus material for future demonstrations, the pus may be mixed with lactophenol on a slide, a cover glass added, and sealed with nail polish.

   b. Microscopically, pus, sputum, or tissue shows large, spherical thick-walled cells or budding cells, 8-20 μ in diameter in direct mounts. Some walls in the cells may be sufficiently thick to look like a double contour or ring. Note organisms in mouse liver (Plate XV).

3. **Cultures:** In order to isolate the fungus, the infected material should be cultured on Sabhi, blood agar or brain-heart infusion agar at 37° C., and on Sabouraud glucose agar or BHI with chloromycetin and actidione at 25° C. Sabhi agar base with chloromycetin is another useful medium at 25° C. Keep 4 weeks before considering negative.

Organisms of the Deep or Systemic Mycoses

COLONY

109 Blastomyces dermatitidis

112 B. dermatitidis colony 37° C

ORGANISMS IN CULTURE

110 Mycelium and conidia

113 Budding cells

ORGANISM IN TISSUE

111 Budding cells in lung tissue

114 Granuloma in mouse—budding cells

PLATE XV

a. <u>Colonies at 37°</u> C. on blood agar or brain-heart infusion agar develop slowly and are cream to tan in color, soft, wrinkled, and waxy in appearance. Conversion from the mycelial phase usually takes 4 to 5 days. The surface of the medium should be moist (see Plate XV).

<u>Colonies at room temperature</u> when first cultured on Sabouraud glucose agar may show a yeastlike growth in early stages of development. Later, coremia or hyphal projections develop on the surface as the so-called "prickly stage," and finally the entire surface becomes downy or fluffy white. Older cultures become tan to brown in color (see Plate XV). Try converting the mycelial phase to the yeast phase.

b. <u>Microscopically</u>, a slide mount from colonies grown at 37° C. show large, round single budding, thick-walled cells similar to those in tissue as well as short mycelial fragments. Check the size of these budding cells.

Slide cultures or mounts from colonies grown at room temperature should show numerous round to pyriform conidia, 4-5 μ in diameter, attached directly on the hyphae or on short stalks. Older cultures have many chlamydospores, up to 18 μ in diameter, with thickened walls (see Plate XV).

4. **Histopathological Studies**: Prepare stained slides from biopsy specimens taken from skin lesions or from internal areas in disseminated blastomycosis. The tissue reaction is usually of the granulomatous and suppurative reaction. The granulomatous type usually has giant cells present with the fungus cells located in the necrotic areas and at times in the giant cells.

The lesions of the suppurative type have a polymorphonuclear exudate with many fungus cells scattered around the tissue or localized in abscesses. Skin lesions may be a mixture of granulomatous and suppurative types.

The fungus cells which are about the same size as cells in the yeast phase at 37° C., vary from 8-20 μ in diameter with double-contoured thick walls and usually single budding forms when reproducing. Each cell is multinucleate.

The organism is readily stained with PAS, Gomori methenamine silver nitrate stain, or Gridley stain. H and E stain will be satisfactory for *B. dermatitidis* in tissue.

5. **Animal Inoculation**: Guinea pigs, rats, mice, or young male hamsters may be inoculated intraperitoneally with infected material from lesions or with saline suspensions, 1 ml of a 1:200 suspension of the yeast phase. Infection should reach a peak in about 21 days, and the animals may die. Intravenous injection of 0.1 ml. of the suspension in mice may produce a rapidly fatal disease.

After autopsy, examine for nodules on the mesentery, omentum, and peritoneal surface. In addition the spleen, liver, and lung area may have nodules that contain the yeastlike budding cells.

Direct slide mounts of pieces of smashed nodules in lactophenol, with the cover glass pressed down to spread the material out, should show the typical thick-walled budding cells. Stained slides may be made from sections of the infected materials. Crushed material from these lesions mounted in lactophenol may be sealed with nail polish for future reference.

6. *Ajellomyces dermatitidis* McDonough & Lewis 1968. Yeast extract agar containing a suspension of pulverized bone meal (15g/l) is used as the medium in a modified block method (McDonough and Lewis, 1968) for study of the ascigerous stage. The cleistothecia are tan in color, 200 to 300μ in diameter, develop thick-walled, closely coiled spiral hyphae that radiate out from a center in the cleistothecium. The spirals form lateral hyphae. Asci with 8 smooth, spherical, hyaline or light tan ascospores, 1.5 to 2.0μ in diameter. This fungus is heterothallic.

7. **Immunology**:

<u>Blastomycin</u>. A skin test with blastomycin, prepared from a culture filtrate, may show cutaneous hypersensitivity in a patient. Positive skin tests are quite reliable although the quality of

the antigen may vary or the level of skin sensitivity may drop or be lost in disseminated cases. Difficulty is encountered from cross reactions, making it necessary to test with histoplasmin and coccidioidin at the same time. (Emmons et al., 1945.) A positive skin test in 24 to 48 hours occurs if the individual is sensitized to the fungus or its products.

a. Antigen preparation: Put 200 ml of the asparagine broth (see section on media) in a liter flask and inoculate with the fungus. After incubating for 30 to 90 days at 24 to 30° C., Seitz-filter, test the filtrate for sterility, and put in vaccine bottles. Dilute 1:100 or 1:1000 and check for potency by intradermal test on people of known hypersensitivity or sensitized guinea pigs.

Knight and Marcus (1958) have shown that polysaccharide antigens from this organism may be as sensitive and more specific than currently used antigens.

Complement-fixation test. This is the most valuable of the serological tests. The yeast form is better to use for preparation of the antigen. The CF test needs further improvement and standardization before it becomes more useful in diagnosis of blastomycosis. The CF titer is low or zero in the early stage of the disease and gradually rises, remaining high in the terminal stage of the disease. After recovery the antibodies disappear. A high CF test and a negative skin test indicates poor prognosis. With a cross-reaction between histoplasmosis and blastomycosis most likely, CF tests should be done at the same time with different antigens (Campbell and Brinkley, 1953).

8. **Special Nutritional Requirements.** The yeast phase requires 37° C. for growth. No special nutrients are essential unless biotin is absent. Less than 0.1 μg per 1000 ml of medium is needed. Organic nitrogen, such as serine or hydroxyproline, increases the amount of growth of the organism. The vitamin and nitrogen requirements are similar for the mycelial phase.

Selected References

1. ABERNATHY, R. S. and D. C. Heiner. 1961. Precipitation reaction in agar in North American blastomycosis. J. Lab. and Clin. Med. 57:604.
2. BAKER, R. D. 1939. The effect of mouse passage on cultural characteristics and virulence for mice of organisms causing blastomycosis. Am. J. Trop. Med. 19:547.
3. BAKERSPIGEL, A. 1957. The structure and mode of division of the nuclei of *Blastomyces dermatitidis.* Canad. J. Microbiol. 3:923.
4. BAUM, G. L. and J. Schwarz. 1959. North American blastomycosis. Am. J. Med. Sci. 238: 661.
5. BENBROOK, E. A., J. B. Bryant and L. Z. Saunders. 1948. A case of blastomycosis in the horse. J. Am. Vet. Med. Assoc. 120:475.
6. BRODY, M. 1947. Blastomycosis, North American type. A proved case from European continent. Arch. Derm. Syph. 56:529.
7. CAMPBELL, C. C. and G. E. Binkley. 1953. Serologic diagnosis with respect to histoplasmosis, coccidioidomycosis, and blastomycosis and the problem of cross reactions. J. Lab. Clin. Med. 42:896.
8. CARMODY, E. J. and W. Tappen. 1959. Blastomycosis meningitis. Report of a case successfully treated with Amphotericin B. Ann. Intern. Med. 51:780.
9. CHERNISSE, E. I. and B. A. Waisbren. 1956. North American blastomycosis; a clinical study of forty cases. Ann. Intern. Med. 44:105.
10. CHICK, E. W., H. J. Peters, J. F. Denton and W. D. Boring. 1960. Die Nordamerikanische blastomykose. Ergebn. Allg. Path. Patholog. Anat. 40:33.
11. CHICK, E. W., W. D. Sutliff, J. H. Rabich and M. L. Furcolow. 1956. Epidemiological aspects of cases of blastomycosis admitted to Memphis, Tennessee hospitals during the period of 1922-1954. A review of 86 cases. Am. J. Med. Sci. 231:253.

12. CONANT, N. F. and A. Howell, Jr. 1942. The similarity of the fungi causing South American blastomycosis (Paracoccidioidal granuloma) and North American blastomycosis (Gilchrist's disease). J. Invest. Derm. 5:353.

13. CURTIS, A. C. and F. C. Bocobo. 1957. North American blastomycosis. J. Chronic Dis. 5: 404.

14. DENTON, J. F. and A. F. Di Salvo. 1964. Isolation of *Blastomyces dermatitidis* from natural sites at Augusta, Georgia. Am. J. Trop. Med. Hyg. 13:716.

15. DENTON, J. F., A. F. Di Salvo, and M. L. Hirsch. 1967. Laboratory-acquired North American blastomycosis. J. Am. Med. Assoc. 199:935.

16. EMMONS, C. W., I. G. Murray, H. I. Lurie, M. H. King, J. A. Tulloch and D. H. Connor. 1964. North American blastomycosis: Two autochthonous cases from Africa. Sabouraudia 3:306.

17. FURCOLOW, M. L., A. Balows, R. W. Menges, D. Pickar, J. T. McClellan, and A. Saliba. 1966. Blastomycosis. An important medical problem in the Central United States. J. Am. Med. Assoc. 198:529.

18. GATTI, F., M. de Broe, and L. Ajello. 1968. *Blastomyces dermatitidis* infection in the Congo. Report of a second autochthonous case. Am. J. Trop. Med. Hyg. 17:96.

19. GILARDI, G. L. 1965. Nutrition of systemic and subcutaneous pathogenic fungi. Bact. Rev. 29:406.

20. GILARDI, G. L. and N. C. Laffer. 1962. Nutritional studies of the yeast phase of *Blastomyces dermatitidis* and *B. brasiliensis*. J. Bact. 83:219.

21. GILCHRIST, T. C. 1896. Case of blastomycetic dermatitis in man. Johns Hopkins Hosp. Rep. 1:269.

22. GUIDRY, D. J. and A. J. Bujard. 1964. Comparison of the pathogenicity of the yeast and mycelial phases of *Blastomyces dermatitidis*. Amer. J. Trop. Med. Hyg. 13:319.

23. GUIDRY, D. J. and F. Maier. 1963. Rapid quantitative method for measuring the sensitivity of *Blastomyces dermatitidis* to fungistatic agents. J. Bact. 85:504.

24. HALLIDAY, W. J. and E. McCoy. 1955. Biotin as a growth factor for *Blastomyces dermatitidis*. J. Bact. 70:464.

25. HARRELL, E. R. and A. C. Curtis. 1959. North American blastomycosis. Am. J. Med. 27: 750.

26. HOWARD, D. H. and R. L. Herndon. 1960. Tissue cultures of mouse peritoneal exudates inoculated with *Blastomyces dermatitidis*. J. Bact. 80:522.

27. HOWLES, J. K. and C. I. Black. 1953. Cutaneous blastomycosis: a report of fifty-eight unpublished cases. J. Louisiana Med. Soc. 105:72.

28. KAPLAN, W. and L. Kaufman. 1963. Specific fluorescent antiglobulins for the detection and identification of *Blastomyces dermatitidis* yeast-phase cells. Mycopathologia 19:173.

29. KNIGHT, R. A. and S. Marcus. 1958. Polysaccharide skin test antigens derived from *Histoplasma capsulatum* and *Blastomyces dermatitidis*. Am. Rev. Tuberc. Pulmon. Dis. 77:983.

30. KUNKEL, W. M., L. A. Weed, J. R. McDonald and O. T. Clagett. 1954. North American blastomycosis - Gilchrist's disease; a clinicopathologic study of ninety cases. Int. Abstr. Surg. 99:1.

31. MARTINEZ-BAEZ, M., A. Reyes Mota and A. Gonzalez Ochoa. 1954. Blastomicosis Norteamericana en Mexico. Mex. Rev. Inst. salub. y enferm. trop. 14:225.

32. Mc DONOUGH, E. S., L. Ajello, R. J. Ausherman, A. Balows, J. T. McClellan and S. Brinkman. 1961. Human pathogenic fungi recovered from soil in an area endemic for N. American blastomycosis. Am. J. Hyg. 73:75.

33. Mc DONOUGH, E. S., L. Ajello, L. K. Georg and S. Brinkman. 1960. *In vitro* effects of antibiotics on yeast phase of *Blastomyces dermatitidis*, and other fungi. J. Lab. Clin. Med. 55:116.

34. Mc DONOUGH, E. S. and A. L. Lewis. 1968. The ascigerous stage of *Blastomyces dermatitidis*. Mycologia 60:76.

35. PROCKNOW, J. J. 1966. Disseminated blastomycosis treated successfully with the polypeptide antifungal agent X-5079C. Evidence for human to human transmission. Am. Rev. Resp. Dis. 94:761.

36. RANIER, A. 1951. Primary laryngeal blastomycosis. A review of the literature and report of a case. Am. J. Clin. Path. 21:444.

37. ROBBINS, E. S. 1954. North American blastomycosis in the dog. J. Am. Vet. Med. Assoc. 125:391.

38. SALVIN, S. B. 1959. Current concepts of diagnostic serology and skin hypersensitivity in the mycoses. Am. J. Med. 26:97.

39. SCHWARZ, J. and G. L. Baum. 1951. Blastomycosis. Amer. J. Clin. Pathol. 21:999.

40. SMITH, C. D., J. W. Brandsberg, L. A. Selby, and R. W. Menges. 1966. A comparison of the relative susceptibilities of laboratory animals to infection with the mycelial phase of *Blastomyces dermatitidis.* Sabouraudia 5:126.

41. SMITH, D. T. 1949. Immunologic types of blastomycosis. A report of 40 cases. Ann. Int. Med. 31:463.

42. SMITH, J. G., Jr., J. S. Harris, N. F. Conant and D. T. Smith. 1955. An epidemic of North American blastomycosis. J. Am. Med. Assn. 158:641.

43. SMITH, J. G., Jr., W. C. Humbert and S. Olansky. 1958. Follow-up blastomycosis sensitivity in an epidemic area. Pub. Health Rep. 73:610.

44. THIRUMALACHAR and A. A. Padhye. 1965. Experimental Blastomycosis treated orally with Hamycin. Sabouraudia. 4:6.

45. THOMPSON, W. F. 1953. Blastomycosis of bone; report of a case. J. Bone Joint Surg. 35:777.

46. WATSON, S. H., S. Moore and F. Blank. 1958. Generalized North American blastomycosis. Can. Med. Assoc. 78:35.

47. WEEKS, R. J. 1964. A rapid, simplified medium for converting the mycelial phase of *Blastomyces dermatitidis* to the yeast phase. Mycopathologia 22:153.

PARACOCCIDIOIDOMYCOSIS

(Parococcidioidal Granuloma, South American Blastomycosis)

Definition:

This disease is a chronic, progressive, granulomatous infection of the skin (Plate XI), mucous membranes, lymph nodes, gastrointestinal tract, and internal organs. The early stages of the infection resemble the symptoms of North American blastomycosis.

Etiological Agent:

Paracoccidioides brasiliensis (Splendore) Almeida, 1930. Synonymy: *Blastomyces brasiliensis* Conant and Howell, 1941.

Occurrence:

1. **Man:** Although most common in Brazil, especially in the state of São Paulo, the disease has been reported in all of South America except Chile, and the area of French and British Guiana. It is also in Central America and Mexico. The organism is apparently introduced into man by pieces of vegetation from contact with soil.

2. **Animal:** No reports of animal infections. Found in intestines of bats.

3. **Soil:** Reported to have been isolated from soils in Brazil.

Laboratory Procedures

1. **Source of Infected Material:** Material from biopsy of lesions, pus from lesions, sputum, or other body fluids would be the most likely material for laboratory diagnosis. Lymph nodes are a good source of the organism.

2. **Examination of Infected Materials:**

   a. Pus or sputum should be placed on a slide using the same procedure as described for North American blastomycosis (page 130).

   b. Microscopically, *P. brasiliensis* appears as single and multiple budding, thick-walled cells 10-60 μ in size. The presence of multiple buds is diagnostic. See Plate XVI.

3. **Cultures:** The infected material should be cultured, following the same methods as given for the isolation of *B. dermatitidis* (under methods of culture).

   a. At 37° C., sealed blood agar cultures require up to 3 weeks before primary isolates appear. Smooth to cerebriform, waxy, cream to tan, yeastlike colonies develop on the surface. Mycelial cultures that are thought to be *P. brasiliensis* should be transferred to an enriched medium, such as brain-heart infusion agar or blood agar, and incubated at 37° C., keeping the surface of the medium moist. Transformation to the tissue phase will confirm identification. (see Plate XVI.)

      At room temperature, the fungus grows slowly on Sabouraud glucose agar, reaching about 2 cm in 3 weeks. The colony may be smooth at first, but later develops short aerial mycelium, white to brown in color. The surface varies from flat, velvety, floccose to partially glabrous colonies to heaped, folded and cerebriform colonies (see Plate XVI).

   b. Microscopically, slide mounts from colonies grown at 37° C., show single and multiple budding cells similar to the tissue form (see Plate XVI). The multiple budding cells, 6 to 30 μ in diameter, have buds 1 to 5 μ in diameter.

Slide cultures or mounts from colonies grown at *room temperature* should show a few round to pyriform conidia 2-3 μ long, attached directly or on short sterigmata. The branching, septate hyphae may have numerous intercalary or terminal chlamydospores, or both.

4. **Histopathological Studies**: Stained slides may have either granulomatous or suppurative tissue reactions similar to that seen in North American blastomycosis. The budding cells may be in the giant cells in the abscesses or scattered in the granulomatous tissue. The budding cell is around 12-20 μ with buds varying from 2-4 or 5 μ in diameter. Some cells may not be in the multiple budding stage or may not have any buds present. The multiple peripheral budding must be present for specific diagnosis.

Satisfactory stains are PAS, Gridley, and Gomori methenamine silver stains.

5. **Animal Inoculation**: It is usually not necessary to inoculate animals for the identification of clinical materials. The disease may be produced by inoculating infected material or a saline suspension of the yeast phase intratesticularly into the guinea pig. After 2 to 3 weeks orchitis develops, and draining sinuses should appear. Pus should be removed for examination on slide mounts. Some strains may produce granulomas or nodular bodies in the mesentery area of mice after about 5 to 6 weeks by intraperitoneal injection of a saline suspension of the organism. The granules may be smashed into thin pieces or frozen sections made and placed on a slide containing lactophenol or other mounting media. Observations are made with a cover glass under the microscope for characteristic budding structures. The frozen sections may be stained.

   a. Try reisolating the fungus in culture from the infected animal.

6. **Immunology**:

   Skin tests have been used in South America (Lacaz, 1956), although the intradermal test is not as useful since the fungus is readily found in the pus by microscopic examination. The antigen, paracoccidioidin, is a sterile filtrate from a broth culture.

   The complement-fixation test is of value because the titer rises as the disease spreads and falls with improvement of the patient. This test is useful in following the course of the disease through chemotherapy. Cross-reactions occur with serum from patients with blastomycosis.

   The Fluorescent antibody test can be specific when sera are used from rabbits immunized with formalin-killed cells. Cross-reactions with some other fungi will occur with sera from rabbits that have been infected.

7. **Special Nutritional Requirements**: Inorganic ammonium salts are good nitrogen sources. Thiamine is stimulatory for the mycelial phase. Organic nitrogen is stimulatory for both phases of the fungus.

Keloidal Blastomycosis (Lobo's Disease)

This disease is characterized by keloidal skin lesions from exaggerated fibrous hyperplasia. The organism, *Loboa loboi,* is abundant in skin lesions and has been difficult to isolate on culture media until recently (personal communication from Dr. C. S. Lacaz). The lesions remain localized in most cases and are without visceral dissemination. The giant cells in the lesions contain the fungus cells, which are characterized by chained pattern of budding.

Organisms of the Deep or Systemic Mycoses

COLONY

ORGANISMS IN CULTURE

ORGANISM IN TISSUE

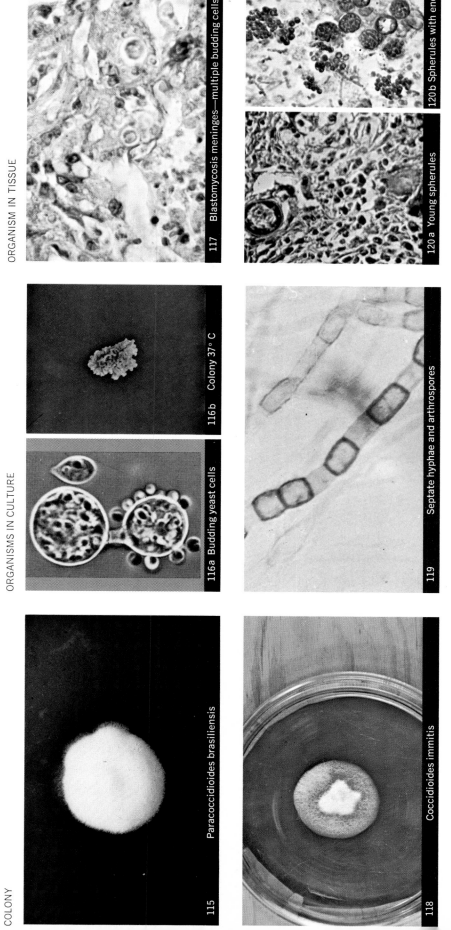

115 Paracoccidioides brasiliensis

116a Budding yeast cells

116b Colony 37° C

117 Blastomycosis meninges—multiple budding cells

118 Coccidioides immitis

119 Septate hyphae and arthrospores

120a Young spherules

120b Spherules with endospores

Plate XVI

Selected References

1. ALMEIDA, F., C. S. Lacaz and A. Cunha. 1946. Dados estatisticos sôbre a granulomatose paracoccidioidica (Blastomicose Sul-Americana ou Paracoccidioidose). Rev. Brasil. Med. 3:91.

2. ALMEIDA, F. and C. S. Lacaz. 1948. Blastomicose "tipo Jorge Lobo". An. Fac. Med. Univ. São Paulo. 24:5.

3. BARUZZI, R. G., C. D'Andretta, S. Carvalhal, O. L. Ramos and P. L. Pontes. Ocorrencia de blastomicose queloideana entre indios Caiabi. Revta Inst. Med. trop. S. Paulo. 9:135.

4. BATISTA, A. C., S. K. Shome and F. M. Santos. 1962. Pathogenicity of *Paracoccidioides brasiliensis* isolated from soil. Inst. de Micol. Public. 373. Univ. do Recife, Brazil.

5. BOGLIOLO, L. 1950. South American blastomycosis (Lutz's disease); A contribution to knowledge of its pathogenesis. Arch. Derm. Syph. 61:470.

6. CIFERRI, R., P. C. Azevedo, S. Campos and L. S. Carneiro. 1956. Taxonomy of Jorge Lobo's disease fungus. Inst. Micol. public. no. 53:1.

7. CONANT, N. F. and A. Howell, Jr. 1942. The similarity of the fungi causing South American blastomycosis (Paracoccidioidal granuloma) and North American blastomycosis (Gilchrist's disease). J. Invest. Derm. 5:353.

8. FONSECA, J. B. 1957. *Blastomicose Sul-Americana.* Estudo das lesnoes dentárias e paradentarias sob o ponto de vista clinico e histopathológico Tése. Fac. Farmácia e Odontologia da Univ. São Paulo pp. 1-182.

9. FURTADO, J. S., T. DeBrito and E. Freymüller. 1967. The structure and reproduction of *Paracoccidioides brasiliensis* in human tissue. Sabouraudia. 5:226.

10. FURTADO, J. S., T. DeBrito and E. Freymüller. 1967. Structure and reproduction of *Paracoccidioides loboi.* Mycologia 59:286.

11. GILARDI, G. L. 1965. Nutrition of systemic and subcutaneous pathogenic fungi. Bact. Rev. 29:406.

12. GILARDI, G. S. and N. C. Laffer. 1962. Nutritional studies of the yeast phase of *Blastomyces dermatitidis* and *B. brasiliensis.* J. Bact. 83:219.

13. GROSE, E. and F. R. Tamsitt. 1965. *Paracoccidiodes brasiliensis* recovered from the intestinal tract of three bats *(Artibeus lituratus)* in Columbia, S. A. Sabouraudia 4:124.

14. LACAZ, C. S. 1956. South American blastomycosis. An. Fac. Med. Univ. São Paulo 29: 1-120.

15. LACAZ, C. S., R. M. Castro, P. S. Minami and A. C. Viegas. 1964. Blastomicosis sudamericana con localización peranal primativa. Tratamiento con anfotericina B. Dermat. Mex. 8:242.

16. MACKINNON, J. E. 1959. Pathogenesis of South American blastomycosis. Trans. Roy. Soc. Trop. Med. Hyg. 53:487.

17. NEGRONI, P. 1966. El *Paracoccidioides brasiliensis* vive saprofiticamente en el suelo argentino. Prensa méd. argent. 53:2381.

18. NETTO, C. F. 1965. The immunology of South American blastomycosis. Mycopathologia 26:349.

19. RAMOS-SILVA, J. 1968. Mise au point sur l'histoire da la blastomycose sudamericaine. Maroc méd. 48:5.

20. RESTREPO, M. A. and T. L. S. Espinal. 1968. Algunas consideraciones ecológicas sobre la paracoccidioidomicosis en Colombia. Antioquia méd. 18:433.

21. SALFELDER, K., J. Schwarz and C. E. Johnson. 1968. Experimental cutaneous South American blastomycosis in Hamsters. Archs. Derm. 97:69.

22. SILVA, M. E. and W. Kaplan. 1965. Specific fluorescein-labeled antiglobulins for the yeast form of *Paracoccidioides brasiliensis.* Amer. J. Trop. Med. 14:290.

COCCIDIOIDOMYCOSIS

(Coccidioidal Granuloma, Valley Fever, San Joaquin Fever)

Definition:

Coccidioidomycosis occurs as a primary infection which is an acute self-limiting respiratory or rarely a cutaneous disease, and as a chronic infection known as progressive coccidioidomycosis (coccidioidal granuloma) which may be fatal, involving the cutaneous, subcutaneous, visceral organs, and bony tissue (Plate XI).

Etiological Agent:

Coccidioides immitis Rixford and Gilchrist 1896.

Occurrence:

The fungus has been cultivated from soil and air in endemic areas.

1. **Man:** Coccidioidomycosis is endemic to the arid southwestern United States. Other areas where the disease has been reported are: Northern Mexico, Honduras, Venezuela, Bolivia, Paraguay, and Argentina.

2. **Animals:** A number of cases have been reported in cattle, while occasional cases have occurred in dogs, sheep and various wild animals including the cottontail rabbit, Townsend mole, European rabbit, mountain gorilla, and the American monkey, and desert rodents.

Laboratory Procedures

1. **Source of Infected Material:** From patients with possible coccidioidomycosis, sputum, gastric contents, spinal fluid, pus from subcutaneous abscesses or exudates from cutaneous lesions should be collected in sterile containers for laboratory examination.

2. **Examination of Infected Materials:**

   a. <u>Direct Examination</u>: Sputum, gastric contents, spinal fluid exudate or pus should be examined directly as a wet mount on a slide with a cover glass. The addition of 10% KOH is desirable if some of the material needs clearing. If a wet mount without KOH is sealed with petrolatum and allowed to remain for 3 to 8 hours, the spherules with endospores will develop hyphae.

   b. <u>Microscopically</u>, round, thick-walled spherules, 20-80 μ in diameter with many small endospores, 2-5 μ in diameter should be found in the infected material. Immature spherules are smaller with a central vacuole (Plate XVI).

3. **Cultures:** Infected material should be isolated at room temperature or 37° C. and cultivated in a well-stoppered bottle or slant containing Sabouraud glucose agar, with or without chloromycetin and cycloheximide. The use of screw-capped tubes may reduce the formation of arthrospores in some strains if semi-anaerobic conditions prevail in the tubes.

   a. <u>The colony</u> develops moderately fast in 3 to 5 days as a moist, membranous gray culture at first, and later develops abundant aerial mycelium, white in color. Older colonies of some strains become more brown in color (Plate XVI).

Some surface areas become glabrous as the aerial mycelium becomes flattened. The diagnostic arthrospores develop in about 2 weeks*.

b. <u>Microscopically</u>, slide mounts with lactophenol and cotton blue, prepared from cultures* containing saline or from killed cultures, should show branching septate hyphae and chains of thick-walled barrel-shaped arthrospores separated by clear spaces, the remnants of empty cells. Older culture mounts show numerous free arthrospores which are in the highly infectious stage (see Fig. 51). The arthrospores are up to 10 μ in diameter.

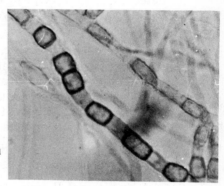

> *NOTE: Special precaution should be exercised in transfer of cultures that contain the highly infectious arthrospores. Saline solution poured into and and flooding the tube near a flame under the hood should help prevent contamination of the laboratory worker. A syringe may be used to insert the saline without removing the cotton plug. The arthrospores are killed readily in 4 minutes at 60°C (Roessler et al, 1946).

c. <u>Culture of spherules</u>: Many culture methods including tissue culture have been developed to produce spherules from the mycelial phase. Reference may be made to articles by Converse and Besemer (1959), Breslau and Kubota (1964), and Northey and Brooks (1962) for more details concerning the media used.

Fig. 51: *C. immitis,* arthrospores in culture, x1200.

4. **Histopathology**: The lesions in coccidioidomycosis resemble several other infections, especially the tuberculous lesions. If stained slides from a biopsy are made or are available for class study, look for the typical spherules with or without endospores, the giant cells, and the granulomatous or suppurative reaction.

The H and E stain may be adequate; however, special fungus stains such as periodic acid-Schiff, Gomori-silver-methenamine, or Gridley stain show more contrast.

5. **Animal Inoculation**: Saline suspensions of arthrospores from cultures or clinical materials may be injected intraperitoneally into the mouse. Between 7 to 10 days the mice should be sacrificed, and the peritoneum, liver, lungs, or spleen examined for lesions or nodules that contain the spherules. By smashing a piece of the nodule or lesion exudate on a slide containing lactophenol and adding a cover glass, the spherules should be visible if the mount is sufficiently thin. Look for different stages in spherule formation including small young spherules, larger ones with vacuole formation, and mature ones with endospores. Other animals readily infected are: rats, guinea pigs, dogs, and monkeys.

a. Stained sections of the infected material from the laboratory animal may be made for pathological studies. Try isolating the fungus from the infected animal.

b. Laboratory animals are useful for immunologic studies related to possible vaccine production that would be suitable for active immunization against this disease.

6. **Immunology**: Much of the information concerning the immunology of the disease has been reported by Smith et al. (1948, 1950, and 1956). The precipitin and complement-fixation tests are useful diagnostic techniques while the coccidioidin skin test is of limited diagnostic value but is of considerable value in epidemiological studies.

a. <u>Coccidioidin for skin tests</u>. Coccidioidin is a filtrate from the liquid culture of the organism. The fungus strains (up to 10 are inoculated into an asparagine broth—see methods section) are grown for 2 to 5 months and filtered with a Berkefeld filter. Merthiolate is added to make a final concentration of 1:10,000. After standardization, coccidioidin is stable at normal temperatures for at least a couple of years (see Smith et al., 1948). Coccidioidin is administered in the same way as the tuberculin test.

A positive reaction in 24 to 48 hours to *coccidioidin* indicates past infection or present infection of the patient. Up to 1½ months may be required before a positive reaction occurs after exposure to the spores, or 2 to 3 days after the symptoms appear. Normally the positive reaction lasts for years except in the final stages of a disseminated case. False positive may occur from cross reactions, especially with histoplasmin and possibly blastomycin.

b. Precipitin test. This is useful to detect the infection before the rise in the CF titer can be detected. The precipitin test can be done in 7 days after infection of the individual, reaching a maximum in 21 days, and then the titer drops gradually. See Smith et al. (1956) for further information.

c. Complement-fixation test. This is the most useful test for diagnosis of progressive coccidioidomycosis. The CF antibodies appear later than precipitins. In primary types of coccidioidomycosis, the CF antibody titer is low until recovery begins, then the titer drops. In progressive types, the titer goes up rapidly and remains high until the patient improves before the titer drops. If the patient shows progressive development of the disease, the titer remains high or rises until near death.

NOTE: For the preparation of the antigen (coccidioidin) for both precipitin and complement-fixation tests reference may be made to Ajello et al. (1958).

7. **Special Nutritional Requirements.** Some strains will form arthrospores more readily on potato dextrose agar. The organism liquifies gelatin, coagulates milk, and can utilize carbon from many sources; however these biochemical reactions are not needed as the characteristic arthrospores and spherules are used for identification.

Questions:

1. Diagram the life history of *Coccidioides immitis,* including both phases.

2. In what way does *Rhinosporidium seeberi* resemble *C. immitis?* Differences?

3. What are similarities and differences microscopically between *C. immitis* and *Geotrichum* sp.?

4. Explain the significance of changes in the precipitin and complement fixation tests during different stages in primary and progressive coccidioidomycosis.

5. What are the similarities and differences in macroscopic and microscopic characteristics in culture and in tissue for *Geotrichum* sp., *Blastomyces dermatitidis,* and *C. immitis?*

Selected References

1. AJELLO, L., K. Walls, J. C. Moore and R. Falcone. 1958. Rapid production of complement fixation antigen from systemic mycotic diseases. I. Coccidioidin. Influence of media and mechanical agitation on its development. J. Bact. 77:753.

2. AJELLO, L., K. Maddy. G. Crecelius, P. G. Hugenholtz and L. B. Hall. 1965. Recovery of *Coccidioides immitis* from the air. Sabouraudia 4:92.

3. BAKER, E. E. and E. M. Mrak. 1942. Utilization of carbon and nitrogen compounds by *Coccidioides immitis,* (Rixford and Gilchrist). J. Infect. Dis. 70:51.

4. BAKER, E. E., E. M. Mrak and C. E. Smith. 1943. The morphology, taxonomy and distribution of *Coccidioides immitis,* Rixford and Gilchrist. Farlowia. 1:199.

5. BASS, H. E., A. Schomer and R. Berke. 1949. Question of contagion in coccidioidomycosis. Study of contacts. Am. Rev. Tuberc. 59:632.

6. BARTELS, P. A., N. Wagoner and H. W. Larsh. 1968. Conversion of *Coccidioides immitis* in tissue culture. Mycopath. Mycol. app. 35:37.

7. BENNETT, H. D., J. W. Milder and L. A. Baker. 1954. Coccidioidomycosis, possible fomite transmission. J. Lab. Clin. Med. 43:633.

8. BRESLAU, A. M. and M. Y. Kubota. 1964. Continuous in vitro cultivation of spherules of *Coccidioides immitis*. J. Bact. 87:468.

9. BROSBE, E. A. 1967. Use of refined agar for the in vitro propagation of the spherule phase of *Coccidioides immitis*. J. Bact. 93:497.

10. BURGER, C. H. and N. F. Levan. 1955. Coccidioidomycosis in the dog. Report of three clinical cases. J. Am. Vet. Med. Assoc. 126:297.

11. CAMPBELL, C. C. and G. E. Binkley. 1953. Serologic diagnosis with respect to histoplasmosis, coccidioidomycosis and blastomycosis and the problem of cross reactions. J. Lab. Clin. Med. 42:896.

12. CAMPINS, H. 1950. Coccidioidomycosis: Un nuevo problema de salud publica en Venezuela. Rev. San Caracas. 15:1.

13. CONANT, N. F. and R. A. Vogel. 1954. The parasitic growth phase of *Coccidioides immitis* in culture. Mycologia 46:157.

14. CONVERSE, J. L. and A. R. Besemer. 1959. Nutrition of the parasitic phase of *Coccidioides immitis* in a chemically defined liquid medium. J. Bact. 78:231.

15. CONVERSE, J. L., S. P. Pakes, E. M. Snyder and M. W. Castleberry. 1964. Experimental primary cutaneous coccidioidomycosis in the monkey. J. Bact. 87:81.

16. EMMONS, C. W. 1942. Isolation of *Coccidioides* from soil and rodents. Public Health Rep. 57:109.

17. FIESE, M. J. 1958. Coccidioidomycosis. Charles C. Thomas. Springfield, Ill.

18. FOLEY, J. M., R. J. Berman and C. E. Smith. 1959. X-ray irradiation of *Coccidioides immitis* arthrospores: Survival curves and avirulent mutants isolated. J. Bact. 79:480.

19. FRIEDMAN, L. and C. E. Smith. 1956. Vaccination of mice against *Coccidioides immitis*. Am. Rev. Tuberc. 74:245.

20. GEORG, L. K., L. Ajello and M. A. Gordon. 1951. A selective medium for the isolation of *Coccidioides immitis*. Science 114:387.

21. HUPPERT, M., E. T. Peterson, S. H. Sun, P. A. Chitjian and W. J. Derrevere. 1968. Evaluation of a latex particle agglutination test for coccidioidomycosis. Am. J. Clin. Path. 49:96.

22. KAPLAN, W., M. Huppert, D. E. Kraft and J. Bailey. 1966. Fluorescent antibody inhibition test for *Coccidioides immitis* antibodies. Sabouraudia 5:1.

23. IZENSTARK, J. L. 1963. Modern travel and coccidioidomycosis. South. Med. J. 56:745.

24. JOHNSON, J. E., J. E. Perry, F. R. Fekety, P. J. Kadull, and L. E. Cluff. 1964. Laboratory acquired coccidioidomycosis. A report of 210 cases. Ann. Intern. Med. 60:941.

25. LANDAY, M. E., R. W. Wheat, N. F. Conant and E. P. Lowe. 1968. A serological comparison of the three morphological phases of *Coccidioides immitis*: complement fixation tests with a pooled antiserum obtained from rabbits with experimental coccidioidomycosis. Mycopath. Mycol. app. 34:289.

26. LEVINE, H. B., J. M. Cobb and G. M. Scalarone. 1969. Spherule coccidioidin in delayed dermal sensitivity reactions on experimental animals. Sabouraudia 7:20.

27. LONES, G. W. and C. L. Peacock. 1960. Role of carbon dioxide in the dimorphism of *Coccidioides immitis*. J. Bacteriol. 79:308.

28. MADDY, K. T. 1954. Coccidioidomycosis in a sheep. J. Am. Vet. Med. Assoc. 124:465.

29. MADDY, K. T. 1954. Coccidioidomycosis of cattle in the southwestern United States. J. Am. Vet. Med. Assoc. 124:456.

30. MADDY, K. T. and J. Coccozza. 1964. The probable geographic distribution of *Coccidioides immitis* in Mexico. Bol. Ofic. Sanit. Panam. 57:44.

31. NEGRONI, P. and R. Negroni. 1963. Estudios sôbre el *Coccidioides immitis*. XV. Su ecologia en la Argentina. Bol. Acad. Nac. Med. [Rio de Janeiro]. 41:493.

32. NORTHEY, W. T. and L. D. Brooks. 1962. Studies on *Coccidioides immitis*. I. A simple medium for in vitro spherulation. J. Bact. 84:742.

33. PAPPAGIANIS, D., E. W. Putnam and G. S. Kobayaski. 1961. Polysaccharide of *Coccidioides immitis*. J. Bact. 82:714.

34. PAPPAGIANIS, D. 1967. Histopathologic response of mice to killed vaccines of *Coccidioides immitis*. J. invest. Derm. 49:71.

35. RIXFORD, E. and T. C. Gilchrist. 1896. Two cases of protozoan (coccidioidal) infection of the skin and other organs. Bull. Johns Hopkins Hosp. 1:209.

36. ROESSLER, W. G., E. J. Herbst. W. G. McCullough. R. G. Mills and C. R. Brewer. 1946. Studies with *Coccidioides immitis;* submerged growth in liquid medium. J. Infect. Dis. 79:12.

37. ROWE, J. R., J. W. Landau and V. D. Newcomer 1965. Effects of cultural conditions on the development of antigens by *Coccidioides immitis* II. Complement fixation and immunodiffusion studies with human serum. J. Invest. Derm. 44:237.

38. SCHUBERT, J. H. and C. R. Hampson. 1962. An appraisal of serologic tests for coccidioidomycosis. Am. J. Hyg. 76:144.

39. SHECHTER, Y., J. W. Landau and V. D. Newcomer. 1967. Disc electrophoretic studies of proteins from *Coccidioides immitis*. J. invest. Derm. 48:119.

40. SINSKI, J. T., E. P. Lowe, N. F. Conant, H. F. Hardin. M. W. Castleberry and J. G. Ray. 1965. Immunization against experimental lethal simian coccidioidomycosis using whole killed arthrospores and cell fraction. Mycologia 57:431.

41. SINSKI, J. T., F. X. Smith and E. P. Lowe. 1968. Survival of dry *Coccidioides immitis* at 4C for five years. Mycologia 60:444.

42. SIPPEL, J. E. and H. B. Levine. 1969. Annulment of Amphotericin B inhibition of *Coccidioides immitis* endospores; effects on growth, respiration and morphogenesis. Sabouraudia 7:159.

43. SMITH, C. E., E. G. Whiting, E. E. Baker, H. G. Rosenberger, R. R. Beard and M. T. Saito. 1948. The use of coccidioidin. Am. Rev. Tuberc. 57:330.

44. SMITH, C. E., M. T. Saito and S. A. Simons. 1956. Pattern of 39,500 serological tests in coccidioidomycoses. J. Am. Med. Assoc. 160:546.

45. TABERT, J. E., E. T. Wright and V. D. Newcomer. 1952. Experimental coccidioidal granuloma. Developmental stages of sporangia in mice. Am. J. Path. 28:901.

46. VOGEL, R. A. and N. F. Conant. 1952. The cultivation of *Coccidioides immitis* in the embryonated egg. J. Bact. 64:83.

47. WINN, W. A. 1963. Coccidioidomycosis and amphotericin B. Med. Clin. N. Am. 47:1131.

48. WINN, W. A. 1965. Primary cutaneous coccidioidomycosis. Arch. Dermat. 92:221.

GEOTRICHOSIS

Definition:

Geotrichosis is a rather rare fungus infection that may produce lesions in the mouth, intestinal tract, bronchi, and lungs.

Etiological Agent:

Geotrichum candidum Link, 1809.

Occurrence:

Geotrichum sp. may be found in the mouth, skin, and intestinal tract of normal people. The more filamentous *Geotrichum* occurs as a contaminant in sputum, cottage cheese, milk, decaying foodstuffs, tomatoes, and in soil.

1. **Man:** There are too few reports to give an accurate record of distribution. Geotrichosis has been reported a number of times in North America and on rare occasions in the Panama Canal Zone, Germany, and Algeria.

2. **Animals:** The disease has been reported in a dog.

Laboratory Procedures

1. **Source of Infected Material:** Sputum, pus, or bloody stools should be placed in sterile containers for laboratory examination.

2. **Examination of Infected Materials:**

   a. Pus or sputum, with or without the addition of 10% potassium hydroxide, should be placed on a slide with a cover glass. Direct examination of bloody feces also may be examined on a slide. A smear of infected material may be stained by Gram method.

   b. <u>Microscopically</u>, the cells of *Geotrichum* are rectangular, 4 by 8 μ, with ends somewhat rounded, or are spherical and 4-10 μ in diameter (see Plate XVII). Stained cells are Gram positive.

3. **Cultures:** Infected material should be streaked on Sabouraud glucose agar plates, with the addition of antibiotics if desired, and maintained at room temperature for 2 weeks or more. Growth is not as rapid at 37° C.

   a. <u>At room temperature</u> the fungus develops rather fast as a flat, membranous or mealy surfaced colony, yeastlike in consistency, white to cream in color (Plate XVII).

   <u>At 37° C.</u> colonies have only a small surface growth and extensive subsurface growth.

   b. <u>Microscopically</u>, the wide septate hyphae segment into rectangular arthrospores, which are variable in size and rounded on the ends. Look for arthrospores that are segmenting on the slide mount (Plate XVII). Germ tubes may be found on one corner of the arthrospore if germination has occurred and is characteristic of *Geotrichum*.

   NOTE: Repeated isolation of *Geotrichum* from a patient is desirable as the organism may be a normal inhabitant or a secondary invader with another disease.

4. **Animal Inoculation:** Infection has not been successful in laboratory animals.

5. **Special Nutritional Requirements:** This organism can assimilate glucose, galactose, and lactose but not Saccharose and maltose. It grows well on ethanol medium. The organism does not ferment glucose, galactose, saccharose, maltose, and lactose.

Questions:

1. Compare the colonial and microscopic characteristics of *Coccidioides immitis* with *Geotrichum candidum*. Any similarities?

2. How does *Geotrichum* differ from common yeasts such as baker's yeast (*Saccharomyces cerevisiae*)?

Selected References

1. HAUSER, W. 1954. Geotrichose der lunge. Ärztl. Wschr. 9:244.
2. KALISKI, S. R., M. L. Beene and L. Mattman. 1952. *Geotrichum* in the blood stream of an infant. J. Am. Med. Assoc. 148:1207.
3. KUNSTADTER, R. H., A. Milzer and F. Whitcomb. 1950. Broncho-pulmonary geotrichosis in children. Am. J. Dis. Child. 79:82.
4. KUNSTADTER, R. J., R. C. Pendergrass and J. H. Schubert. 1946. Bronchopulmonary geotrichosis. Am. J. Med. Sci. 211:583.
5. LINCOLN, S. D. and J. L. Adcock. 1968. Disseminated geotrichosis in a dog. Pathologia vet. 5:282.
6. MINTON, R., R. V. Young and E. Shanbrom. 1954. Endobronchial geotrichosis. Ann. Intern. Med. 40:340.
7. MORQUER, R., C. Lombard and M. Berthelon. 1955. Pouvoir pathogène de quelques espèces de *Geotrichum*. C. R. Acad. Sci., [Paris]. 240:378.
8. ROSS, J. D., K. D. G. Reid and C. F. Speirs. 1966. Bronchopulmonary geotrichosis with severe asthma. Br. med. J. 1:1400.
9. SAËZ, H. 1968. *Geotrichum pseudocandidum* n. sp., isole chez un Cerf d'Eld-Rucervus eldi (Guthrie). Mycopath. Mycol. appl. 34:359
10. SMITH, D. T. 1934. Oidiomycosis of the lungs. J. Thoracic Surg. 3:241.
11. THJOTTA, T. and K. Urdal. 1949. A family endemic of geotrichosis pulmonum. Acta Path. et Microbiol. Scandinav. 26:673.
12. TORHEIM, B. J. 1963. Immunochemical investigations in *Geotrichum* and certain related fungi. I. Introduction and description of the strains. Sabouraudia 2:146.

Organisms of the Deep or Systemic Mycoses

ORGANISM IN TISSUE

123 Organism in sputum

126 Organism in eye

ORGANISMS IN CULTURE

122 Rectangular arthrospores

125 Conidiophore and conidia

COLONY

121 Geotrichum sp.

124 Aspergillus fumigatus

PLATE XVII

ASPERGILLOSIS

Definition:

Aspergillosis may be a localized type infection involving the nail, foot (mycetoma), external auditory canal, or eye; pulmonary type involving the bronchi and lungs; or the disseminated form, which is usually associated with prolonged drug therapy or debilitating diseases. In lung infections a granulomatous, necrotizing reaction usually occurs. In cattle abortion is an important symptom. It is a frequent lung disease of birds. Species of *Aspergillus* may readily invade debilitated patients.

Etiological Agents:

Aspergillus fumigatus (Fresenius) Thom and Church (1926) is the most commonly isolated species. *Aspergillus flavus, A. nidulans, A. glaucus, A. oryzae, A. sydowi, A. niger,* and other species have been reported in some cases as the causative organisms.

Occurrence:

Species of *Aspergillus* are commonly found in soil, farm homes, stables, barns, grain dust, and decaying vegetation. Threshing areas and mills for grinding grain have higher concentrations of spores.

1. **Man:** Aspergillosis is found in all parts of the world. Increasing number of reports of the disease as a secondary infection are occurring following (1) prolonged antibiotic and cortical steroid treatments, (2) debilitating diseases such as carcinoma, tuberculosis, etc., (3) injuries to the subcutaneous tissue and skin or cornea of the eye, and (4) prolonged exposure to cereal grains heavily contaminated with spores of *Aspergillus.*

2. **Animals:** Cow, horse, sheep, pig, cat, dog, rabbit bison, deer. goat, monkey, and guinea pig. The birds include: budgerigar, canary, cormorant, duck, flamingo, goose, grouse, hawk, jay, ostrich, owl, parrot, peafowl, penguin, pheasant, pigeon, rook, seagull, sparrow, stork, swan, thrush, and turkey.

Laboratory Procedures

1. **Source of Infected Material:** Sputum should be collected in a sterile container for laboratory identification. Skin and debris from the ear can be collected in the same manner as given for the dermatomycoses and otomycosis. Repeated sputum samples should be taken. Biopsies may be available for sectioning and culturing.

2. **Examination of Infected Material:**

   a. Sputum should be pressed to a thin film under a cover glass and examined under the microscope. Skin and nail scrapings should be examined in 10% KOH. Granulomatous lesions from birds should be crushed in 10% KOH.

   b. Microscopically, the fungus appears as short fragments of branched, septate hyphae, 4-6 μ in diameter. Conidiophores may be present if sufficient oxygen and space is present in pulmonary cases for growth of these structures.

3. **Cultures:**

   Colonies of *Aspergillus fumigatus* can be isolated readily on Sabouraud glucose agar at temperatures up to 45° C., with antibacterial substances, but not actidione, developing rapidly as white filamentous growths on the surface of the medium, soon becoming green or dark green in color (see Plate XVII). Czapek agar is the medium of choice for identification of the species in case of doubt. Other species of *Aspergillus* that may develop may be identified by referring to Raper and Fennell's The Genus *Aspergillus*. Repeated cultures are important to establish etiological significance.

Microscopically, all species of *Aspergillus* will show conidiophores with large terminal vesicles containing many sterigmata which bear long chains of conidia. The conidiophores may be observed by placing the slant on the side underneath the low power objective of the microscope. Slide cultures will show the undisturbed chains of conidia very well.

a. A direct mount from a colony may be prepared by cutting a thin sliver through the area where conidiophores are forming, placing this sliver on a slide with a drop of 70% alcohol, evaporating the alcohol, and adding a drop of lactophenol cotton blue and a cover glass.

b. *Aspergillus fumigatus* has a smooth-walled conidiophore up to 300 μ in length by 2-8 μ in diameter. The tip enlarges into a typical flask-shaped vesicle up to 30 μ in diameter. Sterigmata are in one series on the upper half of the vesicle with dark-green round, usually echinulate, conidia, 2.5-3 μ in diameter (see Plate XVII). The above characteristics, the bending of the sterigma upward to produce a columnar mass of conidia, and the gray-green colony color are characteristics of the species.

4. **Histopathology**: In bronchial aspergillosis the fungus grows readily in the bronchial mucosa. Conidia and conidiophores may be present. The hyphae are 3-4 μ in diameter with branches and septation.

In disseminated lesions the fungus has occurred in various locations including brain, kidney, myocardium, bone, and skin. In the lungs, necrosis, inflammatory cell infiltration, and granulomatous reaction occur. Colonylike formation may appear at first, later terminated by dichotomous branching. In chronic cases isolated lesions are walled off like a tubercle, the center becomes necrotic, forming a cavity where conidiophores may develop.

If material from a biopsy in humans, or granulomatous gray to yellow nodules from birds, are available, stained sections may be made for study of the histopathological changes (see Plate XVII). The fungus can be demonstrated with Gridley, PAS, and usually H and E stains.

5. **Animal Inoculation**: Animal inoculation is not necessary for the identification of *A. fumigatus* or other species of *Aspergillus*. Experimental infections can be produced in newly hatched birds by exposure to spores, resulting in rapid infection in the air sacs. Pigeons were infected by Henrici (1939) when fed moldy grain. Intravenous injection of a small number of spores in pigeons produced tubercles in various organs.

In rabbits intravenous injection of a spore suspension will produce granulomatous lesions in internal organs, especially the kidneys. Intravenous injection of the spores in mice will produce lesions in the brain and kidney.

6. **Toxins**: Endotoxins produced by *A. fumigatus* are apparently of importance in the acute hemorrhagic lesions that develop when numerous spores are present in birds and animals. It may be the cause of abortions in cattle and sheep if produced by *A. fumigatus*. A potent toxin is produced by *A. flavus* when grown on peanuts. This is of concern when eaten by animals. Many problems are arising from toxins developed in storage of various grains for feeds. Fungi such as *Aspergillus* and many of the Fungi Imperfecti are of concern with this problem. Further current information is listed under mycotoxicoses in the *Review of Medical and Veterinary Mycology* and in the book *Mycotoxins in Foodstuffs* (Wogan, 1964).

Questions:

1. In what ways are *Aspergillus* and *Mucor* similar in tissue? Are there any differences?

2. Why is caution necessary in determining whether *Aspergillus* is pathogenic if *A. fumigatus* is isolated in culture?

3. How does the shape of the vesicle of *A. fumigatus* differ from all other species of *Aspergillus?*

4. Explain under what conditions aspergillosis may be considered a secondary type infection?

Selected References

1. AINSWORTH, G. C. and P. K. C. Austwick. 1959. Fungal Diseases of Animals. Commonwealth Agr. Bureaux. Farnham Royal, Bucks, England.

2. AUSTWICK, P. K. C. and J. A. J. Venn. 1961. Mycotic abortion in England and Wales 1954-1960. Proc. IVth Inter. Cong. An Reprod. The Hague. Pp. 562-568.

3. CHUTE, H. L. and D. C. O'Meara. 1957. A bibliography of avian mycoses. Maine Agr. Exp. Sta. Misc. Publ. 631.

4. CLARK, D. S., E. E. Jones, W. B. Crowl and F. K. Ross. 1954. Aspergillosis in newly hatched chicks. J. Am. Vet. Med. Assoc. 124:923.

5. COON, N. C. and L. N. Locke, 1968. Aspergillosis in a bald eagle *(Haliaeetus leucocephalus).* Bull. Wildl. Dis. Ass. 4:51.

6. EASTCOTT, H. H. and W. H. Hughes. 1963. Postoperative wound infection with *Aspergillus fumigatus.* A case report. Brit. J. Surg. 50:662.

7. EGGERT, M. J. and J. V. Barnhart. 1953. A case of egg borne aspergillosis. J. Am. Vet. Med. Assoc. 122:225.

8. EMMONS, C. W. 1962. Natural occurrences of opportunistic fungi. Lab. Invest. 11:1026.

9. FINEGOLD, S. M., D. Will and J. F. Murray. 1959. Aspergillosis. A review and report of twelve cases. Am. J. Med. 27:463.

10. FORD, S. and L. Friedman. 1967. Experimental study of the pathogenicity of Aspergilli for mice. J. Bact. 94:928.

11. FORGACS, J. 1962. Mycotoxicoses. Proc. 1962. Maryland Nutr. Conf. for Feed Manuf., p. 19.

12. HENRICI, A. T. 1939. An endotoxin from *Aspergillus fumigatus.* J. Immunol. 36:319.

13. HINSON, K. F. W., A. J. Moon and N. S. Plummer. 1952. Bronchopulmonary aspergillosis; a review and a report of eight new cases. Thorax, 7:317.

14. HORA, J. F. 1965. Primary aspergillosis of the paranasal sinuses and associated areas. Laryngoscope 75:768.

15. IKEMOTO, H. 1965. Treatment of pulmonary aspergilloma with amphotericin B. Arch. Intern. Med. 114:598.

16. IVER, S., P. R. Dodge and R. D. Adams. 1952. Two cases of *Aspergillus* infection of the central nervous system. J. Neurol. Psychiat., N. S. 15:152.

17. JANKE, D. 1965. Zur gegenseitigen Beeinflussung von Tuberkulose und Aspergillose. Mykosen, 8:77.

18. KAGERUKA, P. 1967. The mycotic flora of antarctic Emperor and Adelie Penguins. Acta zool. path. antverp. 44:87.

19. KHOO, T. K., K. Sugai and T. K. Leong. 1966. Disseminated aspergillosis. Case report and review of the world literature. Am. J. clin. Path. 45:697.

20. MAHVI, T. A., H. M. Webb, C. D. Dixon and J. A. Boone. 1968. Systemic aspergillosis by *Aspergillus niger* after open-heart surgery. J. Am. Med. Ass. 203:520.

21. MOORE, E. N. 1953. *Aspergillus fumigatus* as a cause of ophthalmitis in turkeys. Poult. Sci. 32:796.

22. PAKES, S. P., A. E. New and S. C. Benbrook. 1967. Pulmonary aspergillosis in a cat. J. Am. Vet. Med. Ass. 151:950.

23. PARADISE, A. J. and L. Roberts. 1963. Endogenous ocular aspergillosis. Report of a case in an infant with cytomegalic inclusion disease. Arch. Ophthal. 69:765.

24. PORE, R. S. and H. W. Larsh. 1968. Experimental pathology of *Aspergillus terreus-flavipes* group species. Sabouraudia 6:89.

25. PROCKNOW, J. J. 1962. Treatment of opportunistic fungus infections. Lab. Invest. 11:1217.

26. RAPER, K. B. and D. L. Fennell. 1965. The Genus *Aspergillus*. Williams and Wilkins Co., Baltimore, Md.

27. STALLYBRASS, F. C. 1963. The precipitin test in human systemic aspergillosis. Mycopathologia 21:272.

28. VALLEJO, L. C. 1963. Aspergilosis pulmonar aguda de los Polluelos. (Neumonia de la incubacion - Neumonia micotica - Neumomicosis). Rev. Med. Vet. B. Aires. 44:321.

29. VEDDER, J. S. and W. F. Schorr. 1969. Primary disseminated pulmonary aspergillosis with metastatic skin nodules. J. Am. Med. Ass. 209:1191.

30. WITTER, J. F. and H. L. Chute. 1952. Aspergillosis in turkeys. J. Am. Vet. Med. Assoc. 21:387.

31. WOGAN, G. N. (Ed.) 1964. Mycotoxins in Foodstuffs. M.I.T. Press, Cambridge, Mass.

32. YOUNG, R. C., C. L. Vogel and V. T. DeVita. 1969. *Aspergillus* lobar pneumonia. J. Am. Med. Ass. 208:1156.

CRYPTOCOCCOSIS

(European Blastomycosis, Torulosis, Buschke's Disease)

Definition:

Cryptococcosis is a subacute or chronic infection involving primarily the brain and meninges, and at times the lungs (Plate XI), skin, skeleton, or other parts of the body.

Etiological Agent:

Cryptococcus neoformans (Sanfelice) Vuillemin, 1901. Some synonyms: *Torula neoformans* Weis, 1902, *Torula histolytica* Stoddard and Culter, 1916, *Cryptococcus histolyticus* Castellani, 1928, and *Debaryomyces hominis* Todd and Herrman, 1936.

Occurrence:

The organism has been isolated as a saprophyte from soil, plants, fruits, milk, skin, feces of normal people, and pigeon dung.

1. **Man:** The disease is worldwide in distribution.

2. **Animals:** The disease has been reported especially in dogs, cats, pigs, horses, foxes, ferrets, cows, cheetahs, monkeys, and sheep.

Laboratory Procedures

1. **Source of Infected Material:** Pus from skin lesions or subcutaneous tumorlike formations should be obtained by aspiration if possible. All material collected, including cerebrospinal fluid, sputum, urine, pus, or visceral organs from autopsies should be put in sterile containers for laboratory examination.

2. **Examination of Infected Material:**

   a. Place a loopful of pus, sputum, urine, or other body fluids in a drop of India ink, mix, cover with a cover glass, and examine for cells with capsules. Spinal fluid should be centrifuged and the sediment placed on the slide with the drop of India ink, then a cover glass added. If the India ink is too dark, dilute to 50% with water. The right microscope light intensity is important for observing the cell and capsule.

   b. <u>Microscopically</u>, India ink mounts of the infected material should show round to oval, thick-walled budding cells, ranging from 5 to 20 μ in diameter. The organisms are surrounded by wide refractile, polysaccharide, gelatinous capsules. Notice that the capsule may be more than twice as wide as the diameter of the cell (Plate XVIII).

3. **Cultures:** Sputum, spinal fluid, blood, or tissues may be cultured on Sabouraud glucose agar. Other selective media are useful including the media developed by Shields and Ajello (1966) and by Vogel (1969).

   Chloramphenicol should be added to reduce bacterial contaminants. Enriched media, such as brain-heart infusion agar, are good for isolation of the organism. The organism will usually grow at both room temperature and 37° C., while saprophytic species usually do not grow at 37°C. Cycloheximide should not be used in the medium as the organism is retarded in growth.

   Shields and Ajello (1966) have developed a selective medium for isolation of the organism from heavily contaminated materials. The medium contains glucose, creatinine, and an extract of thistle seed (*Guizotia abyssinica*) (see page 42 for procedure). Colonies of *Cryptococcus neoformans* assimilate creatinine and absorb the color from the seed extract, resulting in the development of brown color. Other species of *Cryptococcus* and *Candida* grow on this medium without the production of brown color.

Vogel (1969) has developed a selective medium for *C. neoformans*. This is a potato dextrose medium containing urea-antibiotic supplements and a pH of 3.5 (see directions for preparation page 42). Growth on this medium is restricted to *Candida* and *Cryptococcus* species. *Cryptococcus* species develop a moist white colony surrounded by a red halo as a result of the breakdown of urea. No red color will develop if *Candida* species grow on the medium. Incubation of the cultures at 37°C eliminates the saprophytic *Cryptococcus* species.

a. Colonies at room temperature or 37° C. on Sabouraud glucose agar develop slowly and are mucoid, slimy, and cream to brown in color. Primary isolates at room temperatures may be wrinkled and granular in appearance and upon transfer become mucoid. Note the colony in Plate XVIII. Colonies appear in a couple days but mature in a couple of weeks.

b. Microscopically, India ink mounts of a portion of the colony will have thick-walled, ovoid to spherical budding cells up to 20 μ in diameter, with a gelatinous capsule surrounding the cells. The polysaccharide capsule varies in thickness, being up to twice the radius of the cell. In some primary isolates, capsules may not develop until transferred. No hyphae are present (except in rare cases).

4. **Special tests for identification of** *C. neoformans* **(See Table III).**

a. Urease production. Other yeasts or yeastlike fungi, including *Candida* species, do not produce urease, while all species of *Cryptococcus* can produce urease.

Medium. Prepare 100 ml of the Urea Agar Base (Difco) and sterilize by filtering. A second medium containing 15 gm of agar in 900 ml of distilled water is heated to dissolve the agar and sterilized before adding the urea agar base, which should be done when the medium has cooled to about 50° C. The medium is put in tubes and slanted. (Seeliger, 1956.)

Test. A deep red color throughout the medium indicates a positive reaction for urease. Species of *Cryptococcus* produce this color in 1 to 2 days.

b. Nitrate assimilation.

Medium. Prepare a 10X concentration of yeast-carbon-base (Difco) medium, filter to sterilize, and keep in bottles in the refrigerator until needed. Two ml of a diluted suspension of the organism in saline is placed in a plate, 1½ ml of the yeast-carbon-base added and 13½ ml of melted, warm 2% agar is added and rotated to mix well before hardening. An antibiotic assay cylinder is placed in the center of the plate, slightly submerged in the agar, and filled with 1% solution of potassium nitrate.

Test. Species that assimilate nitrates will grow around the cup area in 1 to 2 days at room temperature (25° C.). *Cryptococcus neoformans* is not able to assimilate nitrates.

c. Sugar assimilation.

Medium. Prepare a 10X concentration of a yeast-nitrogen-base (Difco) medium, filter to sterilize, and store in refrigerator until needed. A diluted suspension of the organism in saline is placed in a plate, 1½ ml of the yeast-nitrogen-base and 13½ ml of the warm 2% agar is added and rotated. Up to 6 sterile, antibiotic assay cylinders (small glass cylinders) are flamed and placed on top of the plate. The test carbohydrates, in 20% concentration, are added to fill the cups. Incubate at room temperature (25° C.). Check for colony growth on the test carbohydrates. (Compare with Table III.)

TABLE III

Physiological Characteristics of *Cryptococcus* Species

	C. neo-formans	*C. albidus*	*C. albidus* var. diffluens	*C. laurentii*	*C. luteolus*	*C. terreus*
Growth at 37° C.	+	0	0	+ or 0	0	0
Nitrate Assimilation	0	+	+	0	0	+ or 0
Purine-creatinine	+	0	0	+ or 0 (at 37° C.)	0	0
Sugar Assimilation Glucose	+	+	+	+	+	+
Galactose	+ (weak)	+ (weak)	+ (weak)	+ (weak)	+	+
Lactose	0	+ (weak)	0	+	0	0
Melibiose	0	0	0	+ or 0	+	0
Sucrose	+	+	+	+	+	0
Urease Test	+	+	+	+	+	+

0 = negative
+ = positive

5. **Histopathology.** In tissue sections the organism can be demonstrated with hematoxylin and eosin stain. The most satisfactory stains for demonstrating the organisms are PAS stain, the Gridley stain, or the mucicarmine stain. There is little tissue reaction around the capsules containing budding cells (Plate XVIII). Look for the budding cells in the various types of stained slides if available for study. See references for additional information on pathology of the disease.

6. **Animal Inoculation.** *Cryptococcus neoformans* may be differentiated from other species by pathogenicity tests in mice. About ½ ml of infected material or a saline suspension of the culture should be injected intraperitoneally into the mouse. Intravenous or intracerebral injections is a preferred route. In 2 to 4 weeks, an autopsy of the animal should contain gelatinous masses in the visceral cavity, spleen involvement, and in more virulent strains, infection of the lung and brain. Pathogenicity for mice is correlated with capsular substance (Bulmer and Sans, 1967).

a. Make India ink preparations of the infected tissue or gelatinous mass and look for the typical budding cells with capsules. These mounts are not good after the ink dries and should be sterilized.

    b. Try isolation of the fungus from the lesions in the mouse or rat.

        <u>Intracerebral route</u>. A suspension of a young culture (3 to 5 days old), diluted 1:100 or containing about 100,000 cells per ml, is used for injection. Inoculate the mice intracerebrally with 0.02 to 0.04 ml of the suspension, using a 26-gauge needle. In 1 to 2 weeks the skull may become swollen, and after death, or after autopsy, the gelatinous material from the brain should show budding cells with capsules when put in a drop of India ink.

        <u>Intravenous route</u>. 0.2 ml of about 1,000,000 cells of the organism per ml injected intravenously into mice will usually result in lesions in the brain, lungs, and other organs. Death may occur in 2 to 4 weeks. Intravenous injection of rabbits produces an immediate fever response.

7. **Immunology.** Detection of cryptococcal cells or soluble antigens in sera and cerebrospinal fluid may be determined by the concurrent use of three tests: the latex agglutination (LA) test for cryptococcal antigens, the indirect fluorescent antibody (IFA), and tube agglutination (TA) tests for *C. neoformans* antibodies. This permits a presumptive diagnosis of infections in a high percent of the patients with cryptococcosis (Kaufman and Blumer 1968). For procedures, see Kaufman and Blumer (1968).

8. **Important characteristics used for the identification of** *C. neoformans.* The organism produces capsules, buds, grows at 37° C., does not assimilate nitrates, assimilates glucose, galactose, and sucrose, produces urease, is pathogenic to mice, and in a medium containing creatinine and a seed extract (*Guizotia abyssinica*) produces a brown color, or in potato dextrose medium, containing urea-antibiotic supplements and a pH of 3.5, produces a red halo around the colony. A closely related genus, *Rhodotorula*, may be distinguished from *Cryptococcus* by the usual cartenoid pigments and the inability to utilize inositol.

Questions:

1. How does cryptococcosis differ from blastomycosis in tissue?

2. What are diagnostic characteristics that may be used to differentiate the virulent *Cryptococcus* from the nonvirulent cryptococci?

3. Differentiate *C. neoformans* from *Saccharomyces cerevisiae.*

Selected References

1. AJELLO, L. 1958. Occurrence of *Cryptococcus neoformans* in soils. Am. J. Hyg. 67:72.
2. BARRASH, M. J. and M. Fort. 1960. Amphotericin B in therapy in torula meningitis. Arch. Int. Med. 106:271.
3. BEHMER, O. de A., A. G. Freitas de, and M. D. M. Scalabrini. 1968. Nova técnica para identificacão histoquimica do *Cryptococcus neoformans.* Revta Inst. Med. trop. S. Paulo 10: 124.
4. BENHAM, R. W. 1955. The genus *Cryptococcus:* The present status and criteria for the identification of the species. Trans. N. Y. Acad. Sci. 17:418.
5. BERGMAN, F. 1965. Studies on capsule synthesis of *Cryptococcus neoformans.* Sabouraudia 4:23.
6. BLOOMFIELD, N., M. A. Gordon and F. D. Elmendorf. 1963. Detection of *Cryptococcus neoformans* antigen in body fluids by latex particle agglutination. Proc. Soc. Expt. Biol. 114:64.
7. BULMER, G. S. and M. D. Sans. 1967. *Cryptococcus neoformans.* II. Phagocytosis by human leukocytes. J. Bact. 94:1480.
8. BULMER, G. S., M. D. Sans, and C. M. Gunn. 1967. *Cryptococcus neoformans.* I. Nonencapsulated mutants. J. Bact. 94:1475.

9. CARTER, H. S. and J. L. Young. 1950. Note on the isolation of *Cryptococcus neoformans* from a sample of milk. J. Path. Bact. 62:271.

10. DENTON, J. F. and A. F. Di Salvo. 1968. The prevalence of *Cryptococcus neoformans* in various natural habitats. Sabouraudia 6:213.

11. EINBINDER, J. M., R. W. Benham and C. T. Nelson. 1954. Chemical analysis of the capsular substance of *Cryptococcus neoformans*. J. Invest. Derm. 22:279.

12. EMMONS, C. W. 1951. Isolation of *Cryptococcus neoformans* from soil. J. Bact. 62:685.

13. EMMONS, C. W. 1953. *Cryptococcus neoformans* strains from a severe outbreak of bovine mastitis. Mycopathologia. 6:231.

14. EMMONS, C. W. 1955. Saprophytic sources of *Cryptococcus neoformans* associated with the pigeon *(Columbia livia)*. Am. J. Hyg. 62:227.

15. EVELAND, W. C., J. D. Marshall A. M. Silverstein, F. B. Johnson, L. Iverson and D. J. Winslow. 1957. Specific immunochemical staining of *Cryptococcus neoformans* and its polysaccharide in tissue. Am. J. Path. 33:616.

16. GADEBUSCH, H. H. and P. W. Gikas. 1965. The effect of cortisone upon experimental pulmonary cryptococcosis. Am. Rev. Resp. Dis. 92:64.

17. GORDON, M. A. and E. Lapa. 1964. Serum protein enhancement of antibiotic therapy in cryptococcosis. J. Infect. Dis. 114:373.

18. GOREN, M. B. and J. Warren. 1968. Immunofluorescence studies of reactions at the cryptococcal capsule. J. Infect. Dis. 118:215.

19. HASENCLEVER, H. F. and W. O. Mitchell. 1960. Virulence and growth rates of *Cryptococcus neoformans* in mice. Ann. N. Y. Acad. Sci. 89:156.

20. HOWELL, J. and D. Allan. 1964. A case of cryptococcosis in the cat. J. Comp. Path. Ther. 74:415.

21. KAO, C. J. and J. Schwarz. 1957. The isolation of *Cryptococcus neoformans* from pigeon nests, with remarks on the identification of virulent cryptococci. Am. J. Clin. Path. 27:652.

22. KAUFMAN, L. and S. Blumer. 1965. Development and evaluation of agglutination and fluorescent antibody procedures for the identification of *Cryptococcus neoformans*. Sabouraudia 4:57.

23. KAUFMAN, L. and S. Blumer. 1968. Value and interpretation of serological tests for the diagnosis of cryptococcosis. Appl. Microbiol. 16:1907.

24. KIMBALL, H. R., H. F. Hasenclever, and S. M. Wolff. 1967. Detection of circulating antibody in human cryptococcosis by means of a bentonite flocculation technique. Am. Rev. resp. Dis. 95:631.

25. LITTMAN, M. L. and J. E. Walter. 1968. Cryptococcosis: current issues. Am. J. Med. 45:922.

26. LOURIA, D. B. and T. Kaminski. 1965. Passively-acquired immunity in experimental cryptococcosis. Sabouraudia 4:80.

27. LUTSKY, I. and J. Brodish. 1964. Experimental canine cryptococcosis. J. Infect. Dis. 114:273.

28. MUCHMORE, H. G., F. G. Felton, S. B. Salvin and E. R. Rhoades. 1968. Delayed hypersensitivity to cryptococcin in man. Sabouraudia 6:285.

29. PIDCOE, V. and L. Kaufman. 1968. Fluorescent-antibody reagent for the identification of *Cryptococcus neoformans*. Appl. Microbiol. 16:271.

30. POLLOCK, A. Q. and L. M. Ward. 1962. A hemagglutination test for cryptococcosis. Amer. J. Med. 32:6.

31. PROCKNOW, J. J., J. R. Benfield, J. W. Rippon, C. F. Diener and F. L. Archer. 1965. Cryptococcal hepatitis presenting as a surgical emergency. First isolation of *Cryptococcus neoformans* from point source in Chicago. J. Am. Med. Assoc. 191:269.

32. SALVIN, S. B. and R. F. Smith. 1961. An antigen for detection of hypersensitivity to *Cryptococcus neoformans*. Proc. Soc. Exper. Biol. and Med. 108:498.

33. SANFELICE, F. 1894. Contributo alla morfologia e biologia dei blastomiceti chi sviluppano nei succhi di alcuni frutti. Ann. Isto. Igiene R. Univ. Roma 4:463.

34. SEELIGER, H. P. R. 1956. Use of a urease test for the screening and identification of cryptococci. J. Bact. 72:127.

35. SHADOMY, H. J. and J. P. Utz. 1966. Preliminary studies on a hypha-forming mutant of *Cryptococcus neoformans*. Mycologia 58:383.

36. SHIELDS, A. B. and L. Ajello. 1966. Medium for selective isolation of *Cryptococcus neoformans*. Science 151:208.

37. SWATEK, F. E., J. W. Wilson and D. T. Omieczynski. 1967. Direct plate isolation method for *Cryptococcus neoformans* from the soil. Mycopath. Mycol. appl. 32:129.

38. TAKOS, M. J. and N. W. Elton. 1953. Spontaneous cryptococcosis of Marmoset monkeys in Panama. Arch. Path. 55:403.

39. TRAUTWEIN, G. 1963. Die Kryptokokkose der Haustiere. Disch. tierärztl. Wschr. 70:607.

40. TSUCHIYA, T., S. Kawakita and M. Udagawa. 1963. Rapid identification of *Cryptococcus neoformans* by serology. Sabouraudia 2:209.

41. VANCE, A. M. 1961. The use of the mucicarmine stain for a rapid presumptive identification of *Cryptococcus* from culture. Am. J. Med. Tech. 27:125.

42. VOGEL, R. A. 1966. The indirect fluorescent antibody test for the detection of antibody in human cryptococcal disease. J. Infect. Dis. 116:573.

43. VOGEL, R. A. 1969. Primary isolation medium for *Cryptococcus neoformans*. Appl. Microbiol. 18:1100.

44. WIDRA, A., S. McMillen and H. J. Rhodes. 1968. Problems in serodiagnosis of cryptococcosis. Mycopath. Mycol. appl. 36:353.

45. WILSON, D. E., J. E. Bennett and J. W. Bailey. 1968. Serological grouping of *Cryptococcus neoformans*. Proc. Soc. exp. Biol. Med. 127:820.

Organisms of the Deep or Systemic Mycoses

COLONY

ORGANISMS IN CULTURE

ORGANISM IN TISSUE

127 Cryptococcus neoformans

128 India Ink Preparation

129 Organism in brain—cells with capsules

130 Candida albicans

131 Pseudohyphae, chlamydospore and blastospore

132 a Pseudohyphae, blastospores

132 b Organism in kidney

PLATE XVIII

TORULOPSOSIS

Definition:

Torulopsosis is caused by a fungus that develops as a small (3 to 4 μ) intracellular parasite in tissue and is somewhat like histoplasmosis. It is frequently found in the urine and occasionally in uncomplicated meningitis. It has been reported in the lungs.

Etiological Agents and Occurrence:

Torulopsis glabrata (Anderson) Lodder and De Vries, 1939 in man.

Torulopsis pintolopesii Van Uden, 1952 in the mouse intestinal tract.

Laboratory Procedure

1. **Source of Infected Material:** Human urine, and occasionally sputum or spinal fluid. Intestinal wall of mouse.

2. **Examination of Infected Material:**

   Stained smears or tissue sections show oval to spherical cells, 2-3 μ X 4-5 μ in size, no capsule, no hyphae and no ascospores.

3. **Cultures:**

   Rapid growth on ordinary media. *Torulopsis pintolopesii* requires a temperature of 30° C or above for growth. Sabouraud glucose medium is used for isolation.

   a. <u>Colonies</u> of *T. glabrata* are pasty, white to cream in color at first, later becoming grayish-brown.

   b. <u>Colonies</u> of *T. pintolopesii* develop slowly and are small white or cream colored at 30-37° C.

4. **Biochemical Characteristics:** Both species form acid and gas in glucose. Glucose can be utilized, but not maltose, sucrose, or lactose. Urea is not split or KNO_3 is not assimilated.

5. **Animal Inoculation:** *Torulopsis glabrata* is pathogenic when injected intraperitoneally into mice or rats. Small granulomas form in the animals. The organism develops intracellularly in tissues and must be differentiated from *Histoplasma capsulatum* by cultures.

<u>Questions:</u>

1. How is *Torulopsis glabrata* differentiated from *Cryptococcus neoformans* in culture?

2. How is *T. glabrata* differentiated from *H. capsulatum* in the laboratory animal?

Selected References

1. ARTAGEVEYTIA-ALLENDE, R. C. 1952. Contribucion al conocimiento de *Torulopsis glabrata* (Anderson 1917) Lodder y de Vries 1938. An. Fac. Med. Montevideo 37:470.
2. HAHN, H., F. Condie and R. J. Bulger. 1968. Diagnosis of *Torulopsis glabrata* infection. Successful treatment of two cases. J. Am. Med. Ass. 203:835.
3. HOWARD, D. H. and V. Otto. 1967. The intracellular behavior of *Torulopsis glabrata*. Sabouraudia 5:235.

4. JANSSON, E. 1963. Yeasts isolated from urine specimens. Ann. Med. Intern. Fenn. 52:267.
5. LOPEZ-FERNANDEZ, J. R. 1952. Accion patogena experimental de la levadura *Torulopsis glabrata*. An. Fac. Med. Montevideo 37:470.
6. OLDFIELD, F. S. J., L. Kapica and W. J. Pirozynski. 1968. Pulmonary infection due to *Torulopsis glabrata*. Can. Med. Ass. J. 98:165.

CANDIDIASIS

(Moniliasis, Thrush, Mycotic vulvovaginitis,
Candida perionychia, Candida endocarditis)

Definition:

Candidiasis is a disease with varied manifestations. The acute or chronic infection may show lesions in the mouth, pharynx, vagina, skin (Plate III), nails (Plate II), bronchopulmonary system (Plate XI), intestinal, perianal area, and occasionally endocarditis, meningitis, or infection of other organs.

Etiological Agents:

Candida albicans (Robin) Berkhout, 1923, is usually the pathogenic species in the genus. Some of the synonyms are: *Oidium albicans* Robin, 1853; *Monilia albicans* Zopf, 1890; and *Endomyces albicans* Vuillemin, 1898.

Other species of *Candida* are occasionally pathogenic:

Candida stellatoidea Jones and Martin, 1938, a probably variant of *C. albicans.* This organism usually does not produce chlamydospores.

Candida tropicalis (Castellani) Berkhout, 1923 (Synonymy: *Monilia candida* Hansen, 1888; *Oidium tropicale* Castellani, 1910; *Mycotorula dimorpha* Redaelli and Ciferri, 1935; *M. trimorpha* Redaelli and Ciferri, 1935).

Candida pseudotropicalis (Castellani) Basgal, 1931 (Synonymy: *Endomyces pseudotropicalis* Castellani, 1911; *Monilia pseudotropicalis* Castellani and Chalmers, 1913; *Monilia mortifera* Martin, Jones, Yao and Lee, 1937).

Candida krusei (Castellani) Berkhout, 1923 (Synonymy: *Saccharomyces krusei* Castellani, 1910; *Monilia krusei* Castellani and Chalmers, 1913).

Candida parapsilosis (Ashford) Camargo, 1934 (Synonymy: *Monilia parapsilosis* Ashford, 1928; *M. parakrusei* Castellani and Chalmers, 1934; *Candida brumpti* Langeron and Guerra, 1935.)

Candida guilliermondii (Castellani) Langeron and Guerra, 1938 (Synonymy: *Endomyces guilliermondii Castellani,* 1912).

Occurrence:

Pathogenic species of *Candida* may be isolated from various body sites as a normal saprophyte, ranging from 30% in the oral cavities (Baum, 1960), 38% in the gastrointestinal tract (Van Uden, 1960), 39% in the vaginas (Carter et al., 1959), to 46% in the perianal skin (Recio and DeLeon, 1957). Under certain conditions these organisms may change to pathogens. The organism has been isolated from soil and from fruits.

1. **Man:** Moniliasis is a relatively common mycosis of worldwide distribution. It occurs at all ages and both sexes. There are certain predisposing factors that favor the development of the disease: malnutrition, obesity, diabetes, pregnancy, antibiotic therapy, use of corticosteroids and debilitating diseases.

2. **Animals:** The disease has been reported in chickens, turkeys, ducks, geese, pigeons, pheasants, ruffed grouse, quail, guinea-fowl, dogs, cattle, pigs, colts, lambs, monkeys, hedgehogs, guinea-pigs, and rodents.

Laboratory Procedures

1. **Source of Infected Material**: Collection of infected material for examination will vary considerably depending upon type of clinic symptoms. Skin or nail scrapings, mucous patches from the mouth, vagina or anus, sputum, blood or cerebrospinal fluid or stools may be collected for laboratory study in sterile containers, as smears on slides, or cultured directly. Only freshly collected material is reliable for diagnostic purposes as the organism multiplies rapidly.

2. **Examination of Infected Material**:

    a. Skin and nail scrapings should be mounted in 10% KOH in the usual manner, with a cover glass, and heated gently. Sputum, or mucous material should be pressed to a thin film with a cover glass on a slide. The latter materials may be stained with PAS or by Gram method. The material may also be mounted in lactophenol cotton blue.

    (1) While doing the Gram stain of infected material, or from material provided in the laboratory, try making smears from scrapings in your mouth, especially around the base of an exposed tooth to see if there are any yeast cells present.

    b. Microscopically, species of *Candida* appear on the stained slides or direct mounts from sputum and exudates both as budding cells and fragments of pseudohyphae. The small, oval, thin-walled budding cells are about 2-6μ in diameter (Plate XVIII).

    Since nonpathogenic yeasts may look similar to pathogenic yeasts, special methods of culturing are necessary for identification.

    c. Stools, spinal fluid, or bronchial washings after centrifugation should be examined in the same manner as sputum.

3. **Cultures**: Infected material including scrapings, swabs, sputum, pus, or other materials can be cultured on a variety of media. The addition of penicillin and streptomycin, or chloromycetin and cycloheximide to Sabouraud glucose agar is desirable to reduce contamination in the cultures. The cultures usually grow at room temperature or 37° C. On media containing fermentable carbohydrates, the organism grows primarily as a budding yeast. Without fermentable carbohydrates and with less aerobic conditions along with the addition of more nitrogen in the medium, the pseudohyphae, blastospores, and in some cases, chlamydospores are developed.

    a. Colonies of *C. albicans* on Sabouraud glucose agar appear in 3 or 4 days as cream-colored, smooth, pasty, and have a yeasty odor (see Plate XVIII). Older colonies may have submerged hyphal growth resembling feathers deep in the agar.

    (1) Microscopically, a slide mount will show oval, budding cells 2.5-4 by 6 μ in size and some pseudomycelium if taken from submerged growth. The pseudomycelium consists of elongate, undetached cells with clusters of blastospores at constrictions.

    b. Identification of the pathogenic species *C. albicans:* Ability to produce chlamydospores is usually sufficient to identify this species. If none is present, sugar fermentations and sugar assimilations are useful for species determination. The serum tube method is another useful procedure for identification of *C. albicans.* The presence of numerous yeast cells in blood, urine, or other fluids is significant. Examination of an additional specimen from the patient is desirable to indicate pathogenicity. In sputum the presence of *Candida* species may be significant even in large numbers if another disease is the primary cause.

    (1) Chlamydospore formation. Corn meal agar (including freshly prepared corn meal agar) plus 1% Tween 80, zein agar, rice infusion agar, cream of rice agar, or other types of chlamydospore agars are used for the production of chlamydospores by *C. albicans.* Corn meal, cream of rice, or zein agar with 1% Tween 80 to enhance chlamydospore formation are commonly used media. Chlamydospore formation may be induced to form by direct inoculation of swabs from cases on to Czapek Dox agar after 24 hours (Dawson, 1962).

(a) If a yeastlike colony has developed on Sabouraud agar, transfer onto the surface of the corn meal or other chlamydospore agars. Add a flamed cover glass over the streak. The other species of *Candida* may also be streaked on the same agar for comparison. An identified *C. albicans* may be streaked on the agar for comparison with the unknown. The streak may be made against the bottom of a plastic Petri dish in the medium. Growth can be checked from the bottom under a microscope.

(b) Slide culture technique. Materials include: liquid corn meal agar, plus 1% Tween 80, U-shaped glass tube in a petri dish, slide, cover glass.

Place slide on U-shaped glass tube in petri dish, sterilize. Add warm medium to the warm slide by a pipette or remove the slide and submerge in the medium. Replace the slide after the medium hardens and add water to the petri dish. Streak the surface of the medium and add a flamed cover glass. Incubate at room temperature for 2 or more days and check for chlamydospore formation in the streaked areas under the cover glass. Remove agar medium if below the slide before examination.

(c) Microscopic appearance: under the low power objective, examine the streak on the bottom of the plate or the cover glass on the agar in the petri dish or the slide culture and look for branching mycelium with clusters of blastospores along the sides and the thick-walled round chlamydospores terminating the hyphae. Only *C. albicans* produces the characteristic chlamydospores (Plate XVIII). These are 8-12 μ in diameter.

(2) Serum tube method: The production of filaments or germ tubes by a low concentration of cells of *C. albicans* in serum tubes in 0.5 ml of human serum gives a rapid presumptive identification within 2 or 3 hours at a temperature of 37° C. (Taschdjian, Burchall, and Kozinn, 1960). Make a slide mount at the end of 2 or 3 hours and examine for germ tube formation. Most of the isolates are likely to be *C. albicans* if germ tubes form; however, several other species form germ tubes: *C. stellatoidea, C. utilis, C. rugosa,* and *Schizosaccharomyces fragilis* (Mackenzie, 1962).

(a) A number of factors may prevent the formation of these tubes including too high a concentration of the yeast cells, temperatures above 41° C. or below 31°C., and heat-coagulated serum. Fresh and inactivated human serum, deep-frozen material, as well as dog, rabbit, guinea pig, horse, and bovine sera have proven to be satisfactory.

4. **Sugar Fermentation and Assimilation Tests**: If chlamydospores are scarce, or none are formed, it is necessary to determine the specific pattern for sugar fermentation and assimilation (see Table IV) to determine the species of *Candida albicans, C. stellatoidea, C. tropicalis, C. pseudotropicalis, C. krusei, C. parapsilosis,* and *C. guilliermondii.*

   a. Sugar Fermentation. For each organism to be checked, set up 4 tubes, each containing a solution of one of the following sugars: 1% glucose, sucrose, lactose, and maltose with a fermentation tube in each or covered over with vaseline after the sugars are inoculated. For preparation of the medium see directions under *Media for Specific Use,* page 40.

   b. Sugar Assimilation: For each organism to be tested, prepare 1 or 2 plates according to the directions given under *Cryptococcus neoformans* for sugar assimilation tests, page 156, placing 6 assay cylinders on the medium for the following sugars: galactose, glucose, lactose, maltose, raffinose and sucrose.

5. **Histopathology.** The organisms are not likely to occur in biopsy material unless taken from pulmonary region, mucous membrane of the alimentary tract or bronchi or from endocarditis and systemic cases. Hyphae (pseudohyphae), 3 or 4 μ in diameter, and blastospores (buds) are usually present in tissue in place of oval to round budding cells. The organisms can be readily demonstrated in the Gridley, PAS, or Gomori methanamine silver nitrate stains. H and E stain is satisfactory for demonstration of the organisms in tissue. The demonstration of the organism in tissue is sufficient to designate the genus *Candida.* Study sections containing granulomatous lesions or abscesses.

TABLE IV

Organism	Surface Growth on Sabouraud Broth	Sugar Fermentation				Sugar Assimilation					
		Glucose	Lactose	Maltose	Sucrose	Galactose	Glucose	Lactose	Maltose	Raffinose	Sucrose
C. albicans	0	AG	O	AG	A	+	+	0	+	0	+
C. stellatoidea	0	AG	O	AG	O	+	+	0	+	0	0
C. tropicalis	+ (film)	AG	O	AG	AG	+	+	0	+	0	+
C. pseudo-tropicalis	0	AG	AG	O	AG	+	+	+	0	+	+
C. krusei	+ (film)	AG	O	O	O	0	+	0	0	0	0
C. parapsilosis	0	AG or A	O	O or A	O or A	+	+	0	+	0	+
C. guilliermondii	0	O or AG	O	O	O or AG	+	+	0	+	+	+

0 = negative reaction; A = acid; G = gas; + = growth

6. **Animal Inoculation:** *Candida albicans* and some other species are pathogenic in mice and rabbits. Inject rabbits intravenously with 1 ml of a 1% saline suspension of the organism. In 4 or 5 days the animal should die with abscessed kidneys. For mice, 1 ml saline suspension of the fungus should be injected intraperitoneally, or 0.2 ml. should be injected intravenously. In 7 to 10 days examine the kidney for abscesses. Other species of *Candida* may produce lesions but are usually not lethal.

   a. Prepare sections or smears of the kidney with white abscesses from the infected rabbit or from the infected mouse and stain by Gram method. Look for Gram positive, short, irregularly formed hyphae and budding cells in the section or smear under the immersion oil lens (note Plate XVIII).

   NOTE: Animal inoculations are usually of little diagnostic value in determining the significance of the organism in a patient.

7. **Immunology:** Since *C. albicans* occurs in the intestinal tract, mouth, or vagina of many normal individuals, a positive skin test or presence of agglutinins is of little diagnostic value. Two antigenic groups (A and B) for *C. albicans* have been demonstrated by agglutination and agglutinin-absorption studies (Hasenclever and Mitchell, 1961). Isolates of group A and group B from patients showed little difference in pathogenicity when tested in rabbits and mice (Hasenclever and Mitchell, 1963). Serological identification may be done by fluorescent-antibody techniques with species-specific antisera (after absorption).

Questions:

1. Where does *Candida albicans* occur under normal conditions?

2. What conditions apparently enhance the development of candidiasis?

3. Compare *Candida* sp. with *Saccharomyces cerevisiae.* What are the similarities and differences between these two genera?

Selected References

1. ALKIEWICZ, J. and E. Janiakowa. 1962. A new method of morphological identification of *Candida* species. Bull. Soc. Amis Sci. Poznán, Ser. C, 11:59.

2. BAKERSPIGEL, A. 1962. Sodium taurocholate for the identification of *Candida albicans.* J. Bact. 83:694.

3. BAKERSPIGEL, A. 1963. Chlamydospore production by new strains of *Candida albicans.* J. Bact. 87:228.

4. BAUM, G. L. 1960. The significance of *Candida albicans* in human sputum. New England J. Med. 263:70:

5. BERNANDER, S. and L. Edebo. 1969. Growth and phase conversion of *Candida albicans* in *Dubos* medium. Sabouraudia 7:146.

6. BLYTH, W. 1964. Experimental candidiasis due to *Candida tropicalis:* The effect of oxytetracycline, hydrocortisone and metabolic imbalance. Sabouraudia 3:261.

7. BUCKLEY, H. R. and N. Van Uden. 1963. The identification of *Candida albicans* within two hours by use of an egg white slide preparation. Sabouraudia 2:205.

8. BURROW, M. L. and W. W. Stewart. 1960. *Candida albicans.* Experience with Pagano-Levin culture medium for its identification in clinical material. A report of 294 cultures. Harlem Hosp. Bull. An. Ser. 1:88.

9. DAWSON, C. O. 1962. Identification of *Candida albicans* in primary cultures. Sabouraudia 1:214.

10. DENNY, M. J. and B. M. Partridge. 1968. Tetrazolium medium as an aid in the routine diagnosis of *Candida.* J. Clin. Path. 21:383.

11. FERGUSSON, A. G., N. G. Fraser and P. W. Grant. 1966. Napkin dermatitis with psoriasiform "ide". A review of fifty-two cases. Br. J. Derm. 78:289.

12. FISCHER, J. B. and J. Kane. 1968. Production of chlamydospores by *Candida albicans* cultivated on dilute oxgall agar. Mycopath. Mycol. Appl. 35:223.

13. GORDON, M. A. and G. N. Little. 1963. Effective dehydrated media with surfactants for identification of *Candida albicans.* Sabouraudia 2:171.

14. GORDON, M. A., J. C. Elliott and T. W. Hawkins. 1967. Identification of *Candida albicans,* other *Candida* species and *Torulopsis glabrate* by means of immunofluorescence. Sabouraudia 5:323.

15. HASENCLEVER, H. F., W. O. Mitchell and J. Loewe. 1961. Antigenic studies of *Candida.* J. Bact. 82:574.

16. HEBEKA, E. K. and M. Solotorovsky. 1962. Development of strains of *Candida albicans* resistant to candidin. J. Bact. 84:237.

17. HURLEY, R. 1966. Pathogenicity of the genus *Candida,* p. 13-25. *In* W. I. Winner and R. Hurley (ed). Symposium on *Candida* infections. E. & S. Livingston, Ltd., London.

18. JOHNSON, S. A. M., M. G. Guzman and C. T. Aguilera. 1952. *Candida (Monilia) albicans.* Effect of amino acids, glucose, pH, chlortetracycline (aureomycin) dibasic sodium and calcium phosphates, and anaerobic and aerobic conditions on its growth. Arch. Derm. Syph., 70:49.

19. JORDAN, F. T. W. 1953. The incidence of *Candida albicans* in the crop of fowls. Brit. Vet. J. 109:527.

20. KAPICA, L., A. Clifford and M. Noik. 1969. "Room temperature" incubation for chlamydospore production by *Candida albicans.* Mycopath. Mycol. Appl. 37:338.

21. KEMP, G. and M. Solotorovsky. 1960. Fluorescent antibody studies of *Candida albicans* infections in mice. Bact. Proc. p. 136.

22. KEMP, G., and M. Solotorovsky. 1964. Localization of antigens in mechanically disrupted cells of certain species of the genera *Candida* and *Torulopsis*. J. Immunol. 93:305.

23. KOCKOVÁ-KRATOCHVÍLOVÁ, A., V. Stuchlík and M. Pokorná. 1964. The genus *Candida* Berkhout. V. Basic nutrition of *Candida albicans* in static culture. Folia Microbiol. [Prague]. 9:361.

24. LANDAU, J. W., N. Dabrowa and V. D. Newcomer. 1965. The rapid formation in serum of filaments by *Candida albicans*. J. Invest. Derm. 44:171.

25. LODDER, J. (Ed.). 1970. The Yeasts, A Taxonomic Study. 2 Vol, 2nd Ed. North Holland Publishing Co., Amsterdam, The Netherlands.

26. LOURIA, D. B., R. G. Brayton and G. Finkel. 1963. Studies on the pathogenesis of experimental *Candida albicans* infections in mice. Sabouraudia 2:271.

27. Mac DONALD, E. M. and M. J. Wegner. 1962. A slide culture technique for the identification of *Candida albicans*. Tex. Rep. Biol. Med. 20:128.

28. MACKENZIE, D. W. R. 1962. Identification of *Candida albicans* by serum tube method. J. Clin. Path. 15:563.

29. MACLAREN, J. A. 1961. The cultivation of pathogenic fungi on a molybdenum medium. Mycologia 52:148.

30. MANCHESTER, P. T. and L. K. Georg. 1959. Corneal ulcer due to *Candida parapsilosis (C. parakrusei)*. J. Am. Med. Assoc. 171:1339.

31. MARWIN, R. M. 1949. Relative incidence of *Candida albicans* on the skins of persons with and without skin diseases. J. Invest. Derm. 12:229.

32. MC GAUGHEY, C. A. and A. Bandaranyake. 1953. Moniliasis in guinea-fowl chicks and other poultry. Ceylon Vet. J. 1:43.

33. MEHNERT, B., K. Ernst and W. Gedek. 1964. Hefen als Mastitiserreger beim Rind. Zbl. Vet. Med. 11A:97.

34. MONTES, L. F., T. A. Patrick, S. A. Martin and M. Smith. 1965. Ultrastructure of blastospores of *Candida albicans* after permanganate fixation. J. Invest. Derm. 45:227.

35. MONTES, L. F. and W. H. Wilborn. 1968. Ultrastructural features of host-parasite relationship in oral candidiasis. J. Bact. 96:1349.

36. NEGRONI, R. 1969. Immunologia de las candidiasis. Mycopath. Mycol. appl. 38:190.

37. NICKERSON, W. J. and Z. Mankowski. 1953. A polysaccharide medium of known composition favoring chlamydospore formation in *Candida albicans*. J. Infect. Dis. 92:20.

38. PAGANO, J., J. D. Levin and W. Trejo. 1958. Diagnostic medium for differentiation of species of *Candida*. Antibiot. Ann. 1957. 8:137.

39. REZAI, H. R. and S. Haberman. 1965. The use of immunofluorescence for identification of yeastlike fungi in human infections. Amer. J. Clin. Path. 46:433.

40. SALVIN, S. B., J. C. Cory and M. K. Berg. 1952. The enhancement of the virulence of *Candida albicans* in mice. J. Infect. Dis. 90:177.

41. SCHAMSCHULA, R. G. 1964. The application of the fluorescent antibody technique to the detection of *Candida albicans* in oral pathological material. Aust. J. Exp. Biol. Med. Sci. 42:173.

42. SCHNEIERSON, S. S. and B. Shore. 1965. Adaptation of the Cooper recessed top polystyrene tissue culture dish to identification and investigation of *Candida* and other yeastlike fungi. Applied Microbiol. 13:286.

43. SEBRYAKOV, E. V. 1964. Uskorennaya identifikatsiya *Candida albicans* (Accelerated identification of *C. albicans)*. Veterinariya, Moscow, 41:27.

44. SEELEGER, H. 1955. Ein neues medium zur Pseudomycelbildung von *Candida albicans*. Zeitschr. f. Hyg. 141:488.

45. SELIGMANN, E. 1953. Virulence enhancement of *Candida albicans* by antibiotics and cortisone. Proc. Soc. Exp. Biol. 83:778.

46. SUMMERS, D. F., A. P. Grollman and H. F. Hasenclever. 1964. Polysaccharide antigens of *Candida* cell wall. J. Immunol. 92:491.

47. TASCHDJIAN, C. L. 1957. Routine identification of *Candida albicans:* current methods and a new medium. Mycologia 49:332.

48. TASCHDJIAN, C. L., J. J. Burchall and P. J. Kozinn. 1960. Rapid identification of *Candida albicans* by filamentation of serum and serum substitutes. J. Dis. Child. 99:212.

49. TASCHDJIAN, C. L., P. J. Kozinn, H. Fink, M. B. Cuesta, L. Caroline and A. B. Kantrowitz. 1969. Post mortem studies of systemic candidiasis. I. Diagnostic validity of precipitin reaction and probable origin of sensitization to cytoplasmic candidal antigens. Sabouraudia 7:110.

50. TRIPATHY, S. B. 1965. Observations of changes in turkeys exposed to *Candida albicans*. Diss. Abstr. 25:3187.

51. VAN UDEN, N., L. D. C. Sousa and M. Farinha. 1958. On the intestinal flora of horses, sheep, goats and swine. J. Gen. Microbiol. 19:435.

52. VAN UDEN, N. 1960. The occurrence of *Candida* and other yeasts in the intestinal tracts of animals. Ann. N. Y. Acad. Sci. 89:59.

53. VAN DER WALT, J. P. 1967. Sexually active strains of *Candida albicans* and *Cryptococcus albidus*. Antonie van Leeuwenhock. J. Microbiol. Serol. 33:246.

54. VOGEL, R. A., and R. S. Sponcler. 1970. The study and significance of colony dissociation in *Candida albicans*. Sabouraudia 7:273.

55. WICKERHAM, L. J., C. P. Kurtzman, and A. I. Herman. 1970. Sexual reproduction in *Candida lipolytica*. Science 167:1141.

56. WOLIN, H. L., M. L. Bevis and N. Laurora. 1962. An improved synthetic medium for the rapid production of chlamydospores by *Candida albicans*. Sabouraudia 2:96.

57. WOODS, J. W., I. H. Manning, Jr. and C. N. Patterson. 1951. Monilial infections complicating the therapeutic use of antibiotics. J. Am. Med. Assoc. 145:207.

HISTOPLASMOSIS

(Darling's Disease, Reticuloendotheliosis)

Definition:

Histoplasmosis is a disease involving primarily the reticuloendothelial system. The skin and almost every tissue or organ in the body may be involved. The infection may be localized or generalized. It may be separated into primary histoplasmosis, occurring in the respiratory system, and progressive histoplasmosis with symptoms of emaciation, leukopenia, anemia, ulceration in the nasal region, intestines, and lungs (Plates XI). Liver, spleen and lymph node enlargement usually occurs.

Etiological Agent:

Histoplasma capsulatum Darling (1906).

Occurrence:

The disease, histoplasmosis, is now known to be very common especially in the primary or benign form. Based on skin tests it is estimated that about 30 million people are or have been infected in the United States. About 500,000 new individuals are infected annually. Less than 0.2% develop the progressive form, which has been considered fatal until the use of amphotericin B recently has indicated some promise.

The organism has been isolated from soils, especially around chicken houses, bat guano, or areas used by starlings.

1. **Man:** The disease is more restricted to the Central Mississippi Valley, the Ohio Valley, and along the Appalachian Mountains in the United States. It has been reported in over 30 countries throughout the world in temperate and tropical climates. Histoplasmin sensitivity approaches 80% of the adult population in the Midwestern United States with much lower percentages in other parts of the country. The spores are inhaled from the saprophytic stage in the soil by man and animals for the usual route of infection.

2. **Animals:** The fungus has been isolated from dogs, cats, rats, mice, raccoons, opossums, skunks, foxes, and woodchucks in the United States. Histoplasmosis has also been found in a cow, horse, bat, and African monkey. Positive histoplasmin tests have been reported in cattle, horses, sheep, swine, and chickens.

Laboratory Procedures

1. **Source of Infected Material:** Specimens from peripheral blood, bone marrow, lymph node biopsy, and cutaneous or mucosal lesions should be smeared for staining.

   Sputum should be collected in all cases in sterile containers. One ml or more taken early in the day should be placed in a 0.2 mg/ml of chloramphenicol solution. This should be repeated a few times to determine if pulmonary histoplasmosis can be established. Gastric washings are not necessary unless sputum is difficult to obtain. The containers with the material should be refrigerated until cultured.

   Spinal fluid is taken only if meningeal or cerebral areas are involved and spun down to obtain the sediment for use in culture studies.

2. **Examination of Infected Materials:**

   a. <u>Direct Examination</u>: Peripheral blood smears should be stained with Giemsa, Methenamine-silver nitrate, or PAS stain to examine the material for the presence of the organism.

b. Microscopically, under immersion oil, the fungus should appear as small, round or oval, yeastlike cells, 2-5 μ in diameter, within the mononuclear, or occasionally within the polymorphonuclear cells. Look for these structures in the freshly prepared slides or in the demonstrations for class study. At times cells of *Histoplasma* are found free in the tissue. Giemsa stain shows the cell wall as light blue, with a clear space between the wall and the dark blue protoplasm. Dark oval to crescent-shaped chromatin material appears in the protoplasm. The wall is violet-red to pink with paler colored protoplasm filling the cell if PAS stain is used.

3. **Cultures**: Infected material such as sputum or centrifuged gastric washings should be isolated immediately on several media: Brain-heart infusion with cycloheximide and chloramphenicol at 25° C; on Sabhi agar base plus 10% blood; on BHI agar with 6% blood (no antibiotics), in sealed tubes, at 37° C.; and on Sabouraud glucose agar, at room temperature (25°C.). Cultures should be retained for at least 3 weeks before being considered negative.

a. At 37°C., the yeast growth appears in a few days as a granular to rough, mucoid, cream-colored, round, convex colony turning tan to brown in a couple weeks. Brain-heart infusion agar slants, BHI plus 1% cysteine, Francis cystine blood agar, Sabhi blood agar, and Salvin synthetic medium are satisfactory to maintain or convert the mycelial phase to the yeast phase. Surface moisture is an important factor in the conversion in addition to temperature, medium, and sealed tubes (Plate XIX).

b. At room temperature on brain-heart infusion medium or Emmons' modified Sabouraud glucose agar, two types of colonies may appear from infected material from patients or from soil. The Albino type "A," consists of white, course aerial hyphae while the Brown type "B," consists of flat colonies with light tan to dark brown color in 7 days. Later the brown pigment diffuses into the medium (Berliner, 1968). The white type may become buff color with age. Potato dextrose is a good sporulation medium (for colony appearance see Plate XIX).

c. Microscopically, slide mounts of the yeast phase show oval, or round, small (2-4 μ), single cells with one to several buds. Slide cultures or mounts from colonies grown at room temperature should show septate hyphae with small (2-5 μ), smooth or spiny-walled, round or pyriform conidia borne on short lateral hyphae or sessile on the side of the hyphae. Large (8-20 μ), round to pyriform, tuberculate macroconidia (also known as chlamydospores) are also produced (diagnostic). See Fig. 52, and Plate XIX. The tubercles are 1-8 μ in length. The "A" type produces smooth, or at times tuberculate macroconidia while

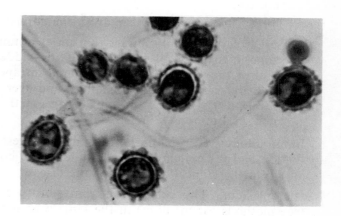

Fig. 52: Macroconidia of *H. capsulatum*, x1200.

the "B" type has masses of tuberculate macroconidia. The saprophytic species of the genus *Sepedonium* produces tuberculate spores like *Histoplasma capsulatum* but no microconidia.

NOTE: The yeast phase should be cultured at room temperature to verify conversion to the mycelial phase and the formation of tuberculate macroconidia (chlamydospores). Conversion of mycelium to yeast phase aids in identification.

4. **Histopathology.** Stained sections of biopsy material should be examined, especially when the organism is not readily found in the blood smears. If stained slides are available, study the pathological changes. Sections through lesions usually show the organisms developing intracellularly in macrophages, and occasionally in giant cells, as the yeast form, 2-5 μ in diameter, surrounded by a capsule (Plate XIX). H and E, Gridley, periodic acid-Schiff technique, or methenamine-silver nitrate stain may be used. The organisms resemble *Leishmania donovani* in size and shape but lack the central nuclear material and the blepharoplast in the stained preparations.

5. **Animal Inoculation:** Mice, guinea pigs, and dogs are susceptible to the yeast phase or spores of the filamentous phase. Mice are the best to use for laboratory studies since they are the most sensitive laboratory animals for isolation of *Histoplasma* from contaminated soil and air samples or from pathological material.

   For sputum add 1 ml of a stock solution containing 7 mg of penicillin and 10 mg of streptomycin per 5 ml (or 0.1 mg of chloramphenicol for each 5 ml of sputum), before injecting intraperitoneally into mice. A pure culture of the yeast phase may be used by injecting 1.0 ml or more of a suspension intraperitoneally into mice for laboratory or class study.

   Sacrifice the mice at the end of four weeks and use the liver and spleen for blood smears and for culture. Hold cultures for one month before considering negative. The intracerebral injection of mice as recommended by Howell (1947), with at least 20,000 or more yeast cells should kill the animals in 7 to 10 days. This may be used as a more rapid method for study of the tissue phase of the organism in class. After autopsy, look for enlarged liver, spleen, and lymph nodes in the animal. Care in handling mice or other laboratory animals should be practiced at all times as feces of mice have been shown to contain the fungus in the yeast phase.

   a. Prepare blood smears from these organs and stain with Giemsa, or periodic acid-Schiff stain. If sections are made of the organs, use stains mentioned under pathological studies. Look for the small, oval to round cells in the mononuclear blood cells using the oil immersion lens.

   b. Try isolating the organism from the animal at 37° C. and at room temperature.

      Soil Isolation. Soil samples that may contain spores of the organism are combined with saline in the ratio of 1 to 5, antibiotics added, the mixture shaken well, and after 1 hour 1 ml of the supernatant is inoculated intraperitoneally into mice. One month later, the mice are sacrificed, and the spleen and liver are cultured on BHI or blood agar (without antibiotics) at 37° C. and on BHI agar with antibiotics in sealed tubes. For further reference see Emmons (1961).

6. **Immunology:** Histoplasmin skin sensitivity tests are useful to indicate the presence or past infection and for epidemiological studies. The complement-fixation test and the precipitin test are an aid in the clinical diagnosis of the disease.

   Histoplasmin: This is a filtrate from a broth culture of *H. capsulatum* grown in asparagine broth (see methods for medium) in the same way as for *C. immitis*. The undiluted filtrate or stock may be stored in the refrigerator for a couple years with dilutions made up with a reference standard. Skin tests with blastomycin and coccidioidin should be run at the same time due to possible cross reactions with related fungus antigens. Positive reactions will occur in 1 to 2 months after infection. Sensitivity in individuals continues indefinitely. A positive skin reaction in 1-to 2-year-old children indicates an active infection is likely, while in older individuals this may indicate past infection. A negative reaction to the skin test may indicate no infection or an early stage of the disease before sensitivity develops.

   Complement-fixation test: Since the sensitivity of the yeast phase antigens are usually greater than histoplasmin antigen but less specific, it has been recommended by Campbell (1960) and others that both antigens be used in tests. The CF titer develops gradually within a few weeks or months after infection. If the patient develops the disseminated form of the disease, this

Organisms of the Deep or Systemic Mycoses

COLONY

ORGANISMS IN CULTURE

ORGANISM IN TISSUE

133 Histoplasma capsulatum

134 Mycelia, conidia, chlamydospores

135 Organism in mononuclear cells

136 H. capsulatum – colony 37° C

137 Budding yeast cells

138 Smear-Mouse liver, PAS, yeast cells

PLATE XIX

will continue to remain high for a long period of time. A second test with a high titer is diagnostic if taken about 1½ months later. In the progressive form of the disease, a high titer usually continues. If a patient improves, the titer gradually falls. Terminal cases may show a rapid drop in the titer prior to death.

Precipitin test: This is of special value in acute pulmonary cases, as a high precipitin titer may occur but no CF antibodies develop. Histoplasmin is used (see Salvin and Hottle, 1948). This test is positive very soon after infection and disappears fairly rapidly.

7. **Special Nutritional Requirements.** The *yeast phase* requires biotin, thiamine, thioctic acid, and sulfhydryl compounds (cysteine) in addition to glucose and inorganic salts in the basal medium for growth factors. The *mycelial phase* utilizes inorganic ammonium as the best nitrogen source with no other special requirements.

8. **Perfect State.** Sexual reproduction in *H. capsulatum* has not been verified at present. *Gymnoascus demonbreunii* (Ajello and Cheng, 1967) was originally considered as the sexual state of *H. capsulatum.* Later it was reported not to be the perfect state (Kwon-Chung, 1968).

African Histoplasmosis

A different type of histoplasmosis occurs in Africa caused by a large form of the fungus, named by Vanbreuseghem, *Histoplasma duboisii.* Over 30 cases have been reported. The granulomatous tissue have giant cells with oval to round thick-walled budding cells, 7-20 μ in diameter. These resemble *B. dermatitidis* in appearance. The mycelial form is similar to *H. capsulatum* in culture. This organism may be a variety of *H. capsulatum* (Ajello, 1968). Larger cells in the yeast phase (Pine, et al., 1964) may be the main cultural difference, while FA antibody staining indicates specific difference (Pine, et al., 1964).

Questions:

1. Are there any other pathogenic fungi that attack the reticuloendothelial system?

2. Differentiate leishmaniasis and toxoplasmosis from histoplasmosis in stained sections of tissue on slides.

3. Compare the similarities and differences of *Histoplasma capsulatum* and *Sepedonium* sp. or *Glomerularia* sp. in culture and microscopically.

4. What cross-reactions may occur with histoplasmin?

Selected References

1. AJELLO, L. 1956. Soil as natural reservoir for human pathogenic fungi. Sci. 123:876.
2. AJELLO, L. 1958. Geographic distribution of *Histoplasma capsulatum.* Mykosen 1:147.
3. AJELLO, L., T. Briceno-Maaz, H. Campins and J. C. Moore. 1960. Isolation of *Histoplasma capsulatum* from an oil bird cave in Venezuela. Mycopathologia 12:199.
4. AJELLO, L. and L. C. Runyon. 1953. Infection of mice with single spores of *Histoplasma capsulatum.* J. Bact. 66:34.
5. AJELLO, L. 1968. Comparative morphology and immunology of members of the genus *Histoplasma.* A review. Mykosen 11:507.
6. AKBARIAN, M., K. Salfelder and J. Schwarz. 1965. Cultural and serological studies in experimental canine histoplasmosis. Antimicrob. Agents and Chemother. 1964:656.
7. BERLINER, M. D. 1968. Primary subcultures of *Histoplasma capsulatum,* I. Macro and micro-morphology of the mycelial phase. Sabouraudia 6:111.

8. BLUMER, S. and L. Kaufman. 1968. Variation in enzymatic activities among strains of *Histoplasma capsulatum* and *Histoplasma duboisii.* Sabouraudia 6:203.

9. CAMPBELL, C. C. 1960. The accuracy of serologic methods in diagnosis. Ann. N. Y. Acad. Sci. 89:163.

10. CAMPBELL, C. C. and G. E. Binkley. 1953. Serologic diagnosis with respect to histoplasmosis, coccidioidomycosis, and blastomycosis and the problem of cross reactions. J. Lab. Clin. Med. 42:896.

11. CAMPBELL, C. C., G. B. Hill and B. T. Falgout. 1962. *Histoplasma capsulatum* isolated from feather pillow associated with histoplasmosis in an infant. Science. 136:1050.

12. CONANT, N. F. 1941. A cultural study of the life cycle of *Histoplasma capsulatum,* Darling (1906). J. Bact. 41:563.

13. DAMLUJI, S. F. and E. A. Kotta. 1964. A survey of histoplasmin sensitivity in Iraq. Bull. Wld. Health Org. 30:595.

14. DARLING, S. T. A. 1906. A protozoan general infection producing pseudotubercles in the lungs and focal necroses in the liver, spleen and lymph nodes. J. Am. Med. Assoc. 46:1283.

15. DOWDING, E. S. 1948. The spores of *Histoplasma.* Can. J. Res. 26:265.

16. EDWARDS, M. R., E. L. Hazen and G. A. Edwards. 1960. The micromorphology of the tuberculate spores of *Histoplasma capsulatum.* Can. J. Microbiol. 6:65.

17. EDWARDS, P. Q. and J. H. Kier. 1956. Worldwide geographic distribution of histoplasmosis and histoplasmin sensitivity. Am. J. Trop. Med. and Hyg. 5:235.

18. EMMONS, C. W. 1949. Isolation of *Histoplasma capsulatum* from soil. Pub. Health Rep. 64:892.

19. EMMONS, C. W. 1958. Association of bats with histoplasmosis. Pub. Health Rep. 73:590.

20. EMMONS, C. W. 1961. Isolation of *Histoplasma capsulatum* from soil in Washington, D. C. Pub. Health Rep. 76:591.

21. EMMONS, C. W., B. J. Olson and W. W. Eldridge. 1945. Studies of the role of fungi in pulmonary diseases; cross-reactions of histoplasmin. Pub. Health Rep. 60:1383.

22. FURCOLOW, M. L. 1958. Recent studies on the epidemiology of histoplasmosis. Ann. N. Y. Acad. Sci. 72:127.

23. FURCOLOW, M. L. and W. H. Horr. 1952. Air and water in the natural history of *Histoplasma capsulatum.* Proc. Conf. on Histoplasmosis, 1952. Pub. Health Monogr. 39:282.

24. FURCOLOW, M. L., W. G. Guntheroth and M. J. Willis. 1952. The frequency of laboratory infection with *Histoplasma capsulatum.* Their clinical and X-ray characteristics. J. Lab. and Clin. Med. 40:182.

25. FURCOLOW, M. L., J. Schubert, F. E. Tosh, I. L. Doto and H. J. Lynch. 1962. Serologic evidence of histoplasmosis in sanatoriums in the U.S. J. Am. Med. Assoc. 180:109.

26. GILARDI, G. L. 1965. Nutrition of systemic and subcutaneous pathogenic fungi. Bact. Rev. 29:406.

27. GOODMAN, N. L., R. F. Sprouse and H. W. Larsh. 1968. Histoplasmin potency as affected by culture age. Sabouraudia 6:273.

28. GOOS, R. D. 1964. Germination of the macroconidium of *Histoplasma capsulatum.* Mycologia 56:662.

29. GONZALES-OCHOA, A. 1959. Histoplasmosis primaria pulmonar aguda en la republica Mexicana. Rev. Inst. Salubr. Enferm. Trop. (Mex.) 19:341.

30. GORDON, M. A. 1959. Fluorescent staining of *Histoplasma capsulatum.* J. Bact. 77:678.

31. GORDON, M. A. and H. B. Cupp. 1953. Detection of *Histoplasma capsulatum* and other fungus spores in the environment by means of the membrane filter. Mycologia 45:241.

32. GRAYSTON, J. T., P. L. Altman and C. C. Cozad. 1956. Experimental histoplasmosis in mice. Pub. Health Monogr. 39:99.

33. HILL, G. B. and C. C. Campbell. 1956. A further evaluation of *Histoplasma capsulatum* in the complement fixation test. J. Lab. Clin. Med. 48:255.

34. HOWELL, A., Jr. 1947. Studies of fungus antigens. I. Quantitative studies of cross reactions between histoplasmin and blastomycin in guinea pigs. Pub. Health Rep. 62:631.

35. IBACH, M. J., H. W. Larsh and M. L. Furcolow. 1954. Epidemic Histoplasmosis and air borne *Histoplasma capsulatum*. Proc. Soc. Exp. Biol. and Med. 85:72.

36. KAUFMAN, L. and W. Kaplan. 1961. Preparation of a fluorescent antibody specific for the yeast phase of *Histoplasma capsulatum*. J. Bact. 82:729.

37. KNIGHT, R. A. and S. Marcus. 1958. Polysaccharide skin test antigens derived from *Histoplasma capsulatum* and *Blastomyces dermatitidis*. Amer. Rev. Tuber. Pulmon. Dis. 77:983.

38. KWON-CHUNG, Kyung J. 1968. *Gymnoascus demonbreunii* Ajello and Cheng: evidence that it is not the perfect state of *Histoplasma capsulatum* Darling. Sabouraudia 6:168.

39. LARSH, H. W., A. Hinton and M. L. Furcolow. 1953. Laboratory studies of *Histoplasma capsulatum*. III. Efficiency of the flotation method in isolation of *Histoplasma capsulatum* from soil. J. Lab. and Clin. Med. 41:478.

40. LITTMAN, M. L. 1955. Liver-spleen glucose blood agar for *Histoplasma capsulatum* and other fungi. Am. J. Clin. Path. 25:1148.

41. LOPEZ, J. F. and R. G. Grocott. 1968. Demonstration of *Histoplasma capsulatum* in peripheral blood by the use of methenamine-silver nitrate stain (Grocott's). Am. J. Clin. Path. 50:692.

42. LYNCH, H. J., Jr., M. L. Furcolow and I. L. Doto. 1962. Therapy of Histoplasmosis in Fungi and Fungus Diseases. G. Dalldurf (Ed.). Charles C. Thomas. Springfield, Ill.

43. Mc VEIGH, I. and K. Morton. 1965. Nutritional studies of *Histoplasma capsulatum*. Mycopathologia 25:294.

44. MENGES, R. W., M. L. Furcolow and A. Hinton. 1954. The role of animals in the epidemiology of histoplasmosis. Am. J. Hyg. 59:113.

45. MENGES, R. W., J. T. McClellan and R. J. Ausherman. 1954. Canine histoplasmosis and blastomycosis in Lexington, Kentucky. J. Am. Vet. Med. Assoc. 124:924.

46. NEGRONI, P. (translated by S. McMillen). 1965. Histoplasmosis. Diagnosis and Treatment. 190 pp. Charles C. Thomas. Springfield, Ill.

47. PINE, L., E. Drouhet and G. Reynolds. 1964. A comparative morphological study of the yeast phases of *Histoplasma capsulatum* and *Histoplasma duboisii*. Sabouraudia 3:211.

48. PINE, L., L. Kaufman and C. J. Boone. 1964. Comparative fluorescent antibody staining of *Histoplasma capsulatum* and *Histoplasma duboisii* with a specific anti-yeast phase *H. capsulatum* conjugate. Mycopathologia 24:315.

49. PINE, L., C. J. Boone and D. McLaughlin. 1966. Antigenic properties of the cell wall and other fractions of the yeast form of *Histoplasma capsulatum*. J. Bact. 91:2158.

50. PINE, L. 1970. Growth of *Histoplasma capsulatum*. VI. Maintenance of the mycelial phase. Appl. Microbiol. 19:413.

51. PROCKNOW, J. J., A. P. Connelly, Jr. and C. G. Ray. 1962. Fluorescent antibody technique in histoplasmosis. Arch. Path. 73:196.

52. ROOKS, R. 1954. Air-borne *Histoplasma capsulatum* spores. Science. 119:385.

53. ROWLEY, D. A., R. T. Haberman and C. W. Emmons. 1954. Histoplasmosis: Pathologic studies of fifty cats and fifty dogs from Loudoun County, Virginia. J. Infect. Dis. 95:98.

54. ROWLEY, D. A. and M. Huber. 1955. Pathogenesis of experimental histoplasmosis in mice. I. Measurement of infecting dosages of the yeast phases of *Histoplasma capsulatum*. J. Infect. Dis. 96:174.

55. SALVIN, S. B. and G. A. Hottle. 1948. Serologic studies on antigens from *Histoplasma capsulatum* Darling. J. Immun. 60:57.

56. SALVIN, S. B. 1949. Cysteine and related compounds in the growth of the yeast-like phase of *Histoplasma capsulatum*. J. Infect. Dis. 84:275.

57. SCHERR, G. H. 1957. Studies on the dimorphism of *Histoplasma capsulatum*. I. The roles of -SH group and incubation temperature. Exper. Cell. Res. 12:92.

58. SHAW, L. W., A. Howell, Jr. and E. S. Weiss. 1950. Biological assay of lots of histoplasmin and the selection of new working lot. Pub. Health Rep. 65:583.

59. SILVA, M. E. and L. A. Paula. 1956. Infecção natural de ratos pelo *Histoplasma capsulatum* na cidade do Salvador, Bahia. Bol. Fund. Gonçalo Moniz. 9:1.

60. SMITH, C. D. and M. L. Furcolow. 1964. Efficiency of three techniques for isolating *Histoplasma capsulatum* from soil, including a new flotation method. J. Lab. Clin. Med. 64:342.

61. SMITH, C. D. and M. L. Furcolow. 1969. Fifteen isolations of *Gymnoascus demonbreunii* from canine and soil sources. Sabouraudia 7:142.

62. SPROUSE, R. F., N. L. Goodman and H. W. Larsh. 1969. Fractionation, isolation and chemical characterization of skin test active components of histoplasmin. Sabouraudia 7:1.

63. STRAUSS, R. E. and A. M. Kligman. 1951. The use of gastric mucin to lower resistance of laboratory animals to systemic fungus infections. J. Infec. Dis. 88:151.

64. SUTTHILL, L. C. and C. C. Campbell. 1965. Feathers as a substrate for *Histoplasma capsulatum* in its filamentous phase of growth. Sabouraudia 4:1.

65. SWEANY, H. C. 1960. Histoplasmosis. Charles C. Thomas, Publisher. Springfield, Ill.

66. VANBREUSEGHEM, R. 1953. *Histoplasma duboisii* and African histoplasmosis. Mycologia 45:803.

67. VANBREUSEGHEM, R. 1964. L'histoplasmose africaine ou histoplasmose causeé par *Histoplasma duboisii* Vanbreuseghem 1952. Bull Acad. Roy. Méd. Belg. 7th Ser. 4:543.

68. WAGONER, N. E., A. L. Morehart and H. W. Larsh. 1965. Improved technique for the reversion of *Histoplasma capsulatum* in tissue culture. Mycopathologia 26:117.

69. WIGGINS, G. L. and J. H. Schubert. 1965. Relationships of histoplasmin agar-gel bands and complement-fixation titers in histoplasmosis. J. Bact. 89:589.

70. WOLPOWITZ, A. and J. Van Eeden. 1963. Histoplasmosis - cave disease. South African Med. J. 37:1002.

71. YATES, J. L., M. N. Atay, H. V. Langeluttig, C. A. Brasher and M. L. Furcolow. 1960. Experience with amphotericin in the therapy of histoplasmosis. Dis. Chest. 37:144.

THE ACTINOMYCETES

The actinomycetes are a group of filamentous microorganisms with some of the characteristics resembling the bacteria and some, the fungi. The group is usually classified with the bacteria in the Class: Schizomycetes. The rudimentary mycelium or mycelium is very thin, being about one micron in diameter, and when fragmented, resembles coccoid or bacillary forms. Some of the organisms in this group are sensitive to the same antibiotics as the Gram-positive bacteria. Other bacterial-like characteristics are: muramic acid in the cell wall structure, the lack of a structural nucleus, and motile forms which are similar in structure.

Since some of the families in the Actinomycetes produce branched mycelium, conidiophores and conidia, the organisms causing diseases are listed among the mycotic diseases. The genera considered in with mycotic diseases which are funguslike are *Actinomyces* and *Nocardia*. It is important to recognize the similarities to bacteria. The term Actinomycete usually includes all of the Actinomycetales except the Mycobacteriaceae. The somatic hyphae or cells are approximately 1 μ in diameter for all members of the group. The order is separated into three families. The Mycobacteriaceae have rudimentary or no mycelium and contain the well-known genus *Mycobacterium*. The second family, Actinomycetaceae, have freely branched mycelium that becomes septate and breaks up into bacillary or coccoid forms. In this family the genus *Actinomyces* is anaerobic or microaerophilic, obligate, and not acid-fast. The genus *Nocardia* is aerobic, partially or nonacid-fast and is a saprophytic or facultative parasite.

The members of the third family, Streptomycetaceae, have well-branched mycelium and reproduce by sporangia or conidia in chains or singly at tips of conidiophores. Spiral conidiophores may be present. The genus *Streptomyces,* containing species that produce most of the commercially important antibiotics, is in this family. This genus reproduces by means of conidia from the ends of hyphae. *Micromonospora* produces conidia singly at the ends of short conidiospores.

The actinomycetes are usually Gram-positive. In smear preparations of the pathogenic forms, the mycelium is extensively broken up into bacillary forms. Colonies vary in the actinomycetes. A wide variety of nitrogen and carbon compounds can be utilized, and many show proteolytic activity. Differentiation of species of the actinomycetes is based on morphological and physiological characteristics.

ACTINOMYCOSIS

Definition:

Actinomycosis is a chronic suppurative and granulomatous fungus infection with lesions or draining sinuses discharging the characteristic "sulfur granules." The disease is more common in the head and neck but may spread to the abdominal organs, thoracic organs, and other parts of the body (Plate XI).

Etiological Agents

Actinomyces israelii (Harz) Kruse, 1896 (Synonymy: *Discomyces bovis* Rivolta, 1878; *Nocardia actinomyces* Trev., 1889; *Cladothrix bovis* Mace, 1891) is the usual organism isolated from human lesions or from normal human tissues.

Actinomyces eriksonii Georg, Roberstad, Brinkman and Hicklin, 1965. A few human cases.

Actinomyces naeslundii Thompson and Lovestedt, 1951. Reported as nonpathogenic in man.

Actinomyces bovis Harz, 1877. (Synonyms are: *Actinomyces israelii* Larchner-Sandoval, 1898; *Streptothrix bovis* Chester, 1901; and *Nocardia bovis* Blanchard, 1896 is usually isolated from bovine sources (Pine, Howell, and Watson, 1960).

Occurrence:

Actinomyces israelii has been isolated from the surface of carious teeth, tonsillar crypts, various areas of the mouth, and sputum by various investigators (Emmons, 1938, Rosebury et al., 1944). The organism has not been isolated from soil or plant sources. Frost (1940) reported *A. bovis* from the mouths of normal cattle. The endogenous origin for both organisms is indicated with the main locations being in the tonsillar crypts and the teeth.

1. **Man:** Actinomycosis is worldwide in occurrence.
2. **Animals:** Most of the cases have been reported in turkeys, cattle, sheep, pigs, dogs, horses, deer, and cats.

Laboratory Procedures

1. **Source of Infected Material:** Pus should be collected in a sterile container (test tube or bottle) as it drains out of sinus or be removed from unopened lesions with a syringe. Sputum, urine, biopsy or autopsy material may be available for laboratory examination.

2. **Examination of Infected Material:**

   a. Place a loopful of pus containing one or more "sulfur granules" on a slide, and lightly crush it with a cover glass. Eosin may be added to the pus to color the granules. Another granule should be smeared on a slide and stained by the Gram method.

   b. Microscopically, the unstained granule is composed of fine, branching, interwoven hyphae (1 μ in diameter). In some strains the ends of the hyphae are frequently surrounded by gelatinous sheaths which give the appearance of club-shaped structures around the edges of the granule. The granule is apparently cemented together by a polysaccharide-protein complex containing about 50% calcium phosphate (Pine and Overman, 1963). On the Gram-stained slide, under immersion oil lens, note the Gram-positive branched hyphae (see Plate X). Some old hyphae may be short, rod-shaped, bacterial-like, and appear Gram-negative.

   If material contains no granules, then the pus or sputum from cases considered possible actinomycosis should be smeared, stained, and examined for Gram-positive branched hyphal forms.

Actinomycosis

ORGANISM IN TISSUE

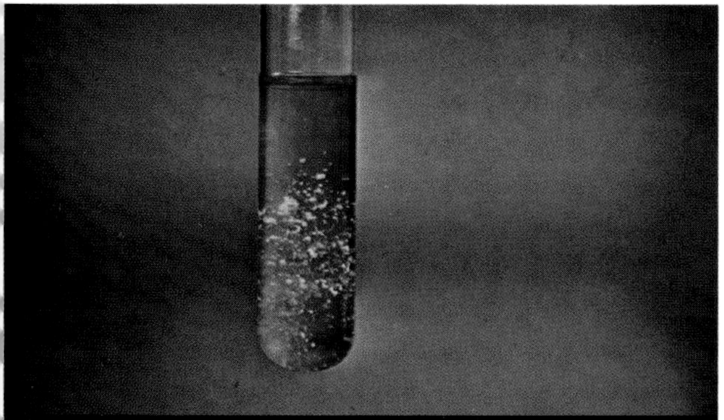

141 b (h.p.f. shows clubs)

141 a   Sulfur granule

Granule—in cow

144

ORGANISMS IN CULTURE

Mycelium-gram stain

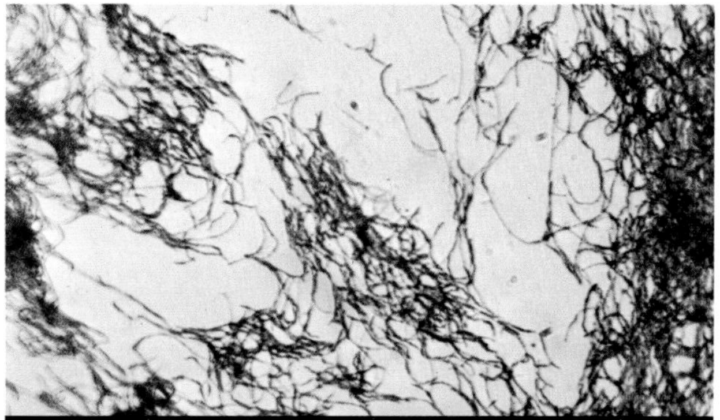

140

Mycelium-gram stain

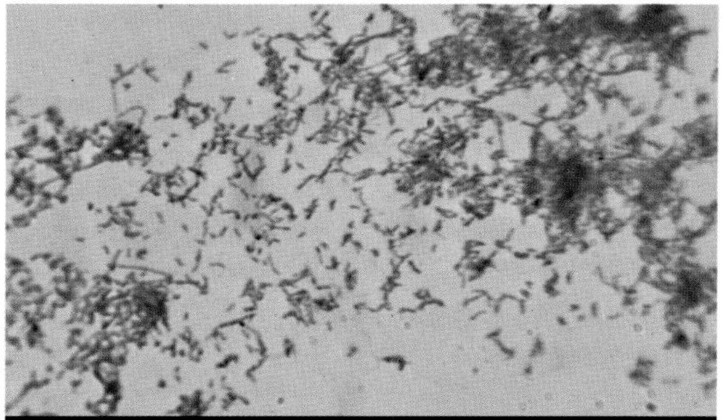

143

PLATE XX

COLONY

Actinomyces israelii-thioglycolate

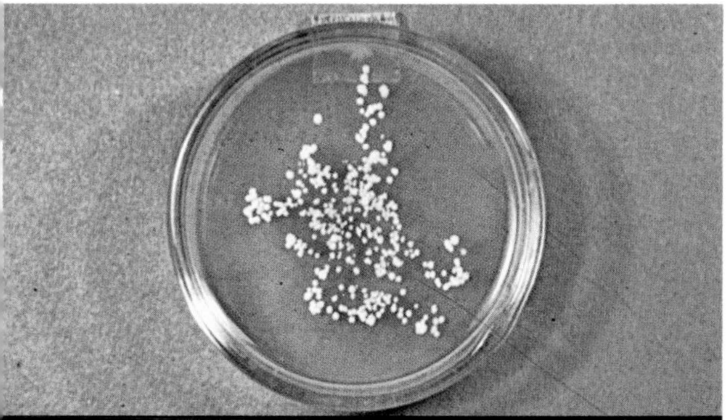

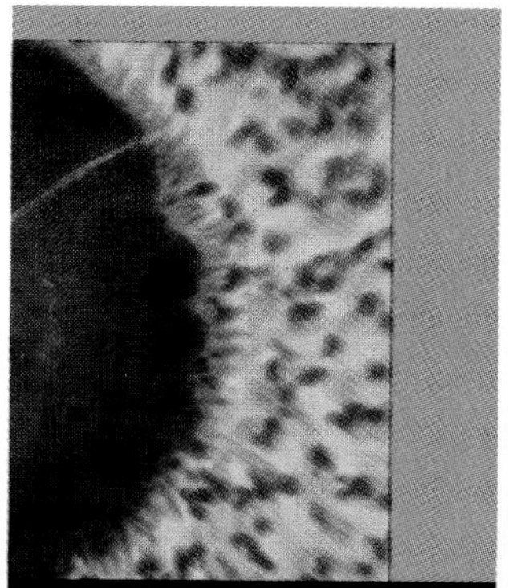

139

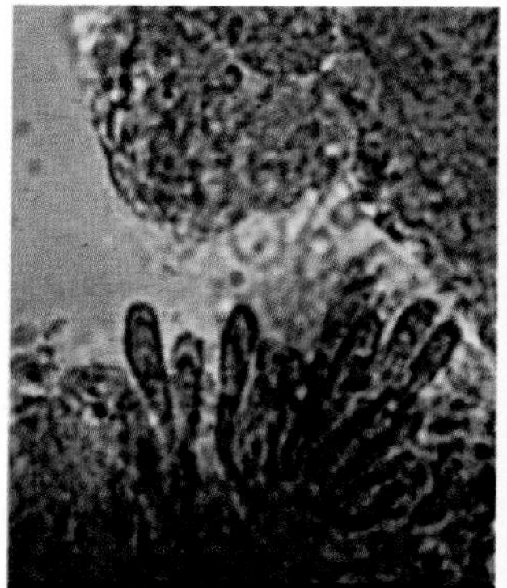

Actinomyces bovis: brain-heart infusion

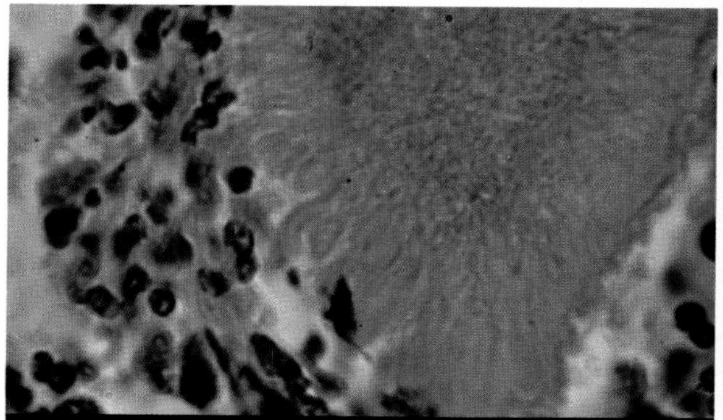

142

If the acid-fast stain is made, the organisms will show nonacid-fast branched forms.

3. **Cultures**: Gram-positive, nonacid-fast branching hyphal forms from granules or from cases without granules should be cultured under anaerobic conditions. All *Actinomyces* sp. are anaerobic and catalase negative. If the material is uncontaminated, the organisms can be grown in Thioglycollate broth, deep shake cultures of beef infusion glucose agar, or chopped meat medium sealed up for anaerobic conditions at 37°C. In 4 to 5 days colonies appear about 1.5 cm below the surface of the medium (Plate XX).

Contaminated material should be washed several times in sterile distilled water to remove contaminating organisms before crushing the granules and streaking on the agar surface. A number of media may be used for isolation of species of *Actinomyces:* brain-heart infusion agar, BHI with 10% rabbit blood, BHI with 0.2% glucose, casitone-starch medium (Howell and Pine). The appearance of the colonies on BHI at the end of about 7 days and a negative catalase test are important in identification of the species (Plate XX). The above culture media should be incubated at 37°C under 95% nitrogen and 5% CO_2 for 5 to 7 days.

The transfer of colonies resembling *A. israelii, A. eriksonii,* or *A. bovis* to broth culture is useful to show the characteristic growth pattern. Branching forms are usually abundant. Colonies appear in 4 to 6 days about 5 mm below the surface, with the broth remaining clear. The saprophytic species, *A. naeslundii* grows and spreads rapidly throughout the medium.

a. <u>Colonies</u>. On streaked plates, the colonies appear as a small, white, smooth to rough convex surface, with a fuzzy or smooth edge, depending on the species. The colonies develop in 7 to 10 days.

b. <u>Microscopically</u>, colonies crushed in a drop of water on a slide with a cover glass show tangled masses of branching hyphae 1 μ in diameter, as seen in Plate XX. Stained smears show Gram-positive branching hyphae and/or pleomorphic diphtheroidlike rods, depending upon species.

c. <u>Identification of species of Actinomyces based on morphological and physiological characteristics</u>. Two references by Georg et al., (1964, 1965) separate the microaerophilic and anaerobic *Actinomyces* species on the basis of morphological, biochemical, and immunological differences. Reference should be made to these papers for detailed information. Some of the distinguishing features are given in the tables following. (see Tables V, VI).

The physiological characteristics including biochemical tests are useful in the separation of species of *Actinomyces. Actinomyces eriksonii* resembles morphologically, but differs from *A. israelii* and *naeslundii* in biochemical reactions, and oxygen requirements (see Table VI). The agar gel precipitin reactions are reported by Georg et al. (1965) to be antigenically distinct for *A. eriksonii.*

(1) <u>Media for Biochemical Tests</u>.

    (a) <u>Catalase Test</u>. A small amount of the colony is placed on a slide, and a drop of peroxide (fresh H_2O_2) is added. No bubble formation should occur for the *Actinomyces* species (negative).

    (b) <u>Gelatin Liquefaction</u>. Check the gelatin liquefaction reaction on gelatin-heart infusion casitone medium (see page 38 for preparation). Use pyrogallol-carbonate seal (see page 38), incubate 4 weeks at 37°C.

    (c) <u>Litmus Milk</u>. Inoculate the medium, add the pyrogallol-carbonate seals on the cotton plugs and incubate for 4 weeks at 37°C. For preparation of medium see page 38.

    (d) <u>Nitrate Reduction</u>. Inoculate the medium, add pyrogallol-carbonate seals, and incubate at 37°C. Test small amounts 2 or 3 times during a two-week interval for nitrate reaction (a few drops of both sulfanilic acid solution [glacial acetic acid, 100 ml; water, 250 ml; sulfanilic acid, 2.8 g], and dimethyl-alpha-naphthylamine solution [glacial acetic acid, 100 ml; water 250 ml; dimethyl-alpha-naphthylamine, 2.1

ml]), which should show a red to brown color, if nitrates are reduced to nitrites. Zinc may be used to reduce the remaining nitrates or see if the organisms did not reduce nitrates.

(e) <u>Starch Hydrolysis</u>. Use plates or tubes of casitone starch medium (see section on "Media for Specific Use," page 37) and streak the culture on the surface. Use an anaerobic jar for plates or seal the tubes with the pyrogallol-carbonate seal, and maintain at 37° C. Test the surface at the end of 5 or 10 days with Gram iodine. A clear area around the colony indicates hydrolysis, and deep blue would mean no hydrolysis.

(f) <u>Sugar Fermentations</u>. After the organism has been growing in heart infusion broth (or sugar-free medium), transfer to sugar fermentation tubes and seal with pyrogallol-carbonate seals. Incubate for 1 month at 37° C., checking for acid formation periodically. See page 38 for preparation of medium.

TABLE Ⅴ
Morphological Characteristics

Characteristic	A. israelii	A. bovis	A. eriksonii*	A. naeslundii
Colonies on BHI Agar 7-10 days 37° C.	Rough colony (R form) starts as "spider" or granularlike with lacelike border. Later lobulate, molar-tooth glistening colony. "S" or smooth form transparent, like A. bovis.	Dewdroplike then entire edge, convex, cream color (S forms). Rare R forms resemble A. israelii, with scalloped border, lumpy surface.	Similar to A. bovis; white to cream, convex to conical, smooth or pebbly surfaced with scalloped edge.	Colonies similar to A. bovis or A. israelii, Smooth "S" forms most common.
Colonies in Thioglycollate Broth, 37° C.	Rough lobulate, or with fuzzy edges, broth clear, colonies not broken readily.	Soft, diffuse colonies, or crumblike colonies, break-up readily.	Soft, lobular colonies, diffuse growth, broth cloudy if shaken.	Fast grower, granular or floccose colonies, diffuse, somewhat cloudy.
Microscopic (All Gram-positive)	Rods and branched forms, some with clubbed ends. Long hyphae at times. Diptheroid in "S" form.	Diptheroid forms usual, branching rare. The rare "R" strains with long branched hyphae.	Straight or curved rods. Usually diptheroidal, some filamentous and branched, clubbed ends present.	Short hyphae with branches, irregular, long hyphae vary in thickness. Some diphtheroidlike forms.

*From Georg et al., (1965).

TABLE VI

Physiological Characteristics

Reactions (37° C.)	A. israelii	A. bovis	A. eriksonii*	A. naeslundii
O_2 Requirements	anaerobic to microaerophilic	Anaerobic to microaerophilic	Obligate anaerobe	Facultative with increased CO_2 present
(Biochemical)				
Catalase	0	0.	0	0
Gelatin liquefaction	0	0	0	0
Litmus milk reaction	Reduced	Reduced	Reduced and firm curd	Reduced and firm curd
Nitrate reduction	+ (80%)	0	0	+ (90%)
Starch hydrolysis	0 (usually)	4 +	4 +	0 (usually)
Sugar Fermentation (Acid formation only)				
Glucose	+	+	+	+
Mannitol	+ (80%)	0	+	0
Mannose	+	0 or ±	+	+
Raffinose	Varies	0	+	+ (80%)
Xylose	+ (80%)	0	+	0

*From Georg et al., (1965).

4. **Histopathology.** If material is available from biopsy, prepare sections, and stain with H and E, PAS, or Gridley stains for showing the granules. The use of Gram stain or Gomori-methenamine silver stain will bring out the mycelium better and not the granules.

Microscopically these sections or other prepared slides will show variations in appearance of the lesions from an abscess with polymorphonuclear cells to proliferation of connective tissue.

Commonly found in histological sections are many leukocytes in necrotic areas surrounded with granulation tissue. The granule usually has well-branched mycelium loosely or compactly formed, with or without clubs on the surface of the granule. The "sulfur granule" is characteristic of some, but not all, species of *Actinomyces*. Cultures are necessary to determine the causative agent.

NOTE: The demonstration of the typical sulfur granule in tissue or pus of a specimen is sufficient to indicate the diagnosis of actinomycosis in man. In cattle actinomycosis and actinobacillosis can be differentiated on a Gram-stained smear, as *Actinomyces* has Gram-positive diphtheroidlike fragments while actinobacilli is Gram-negative.

5. **Animal Inoculation**: Occasional pathogenicity has been established in male hamsters and mice with *A. bovis*. The procedures are not very satisfactory for class demonstrations of the disease. Hazen *et al.*, (1958) have produced infection in hamsters intraperitoneally injected with pure cultures. Meyer and Verges (1950) demonstrated progressive infection of actinomycosis in young mice injected with cultures suspended in 5% gastric mucin (hog).

At the end of 4 weeks the hamsters are checked for external lesions and autopsied. Pus from internal abscesses should be examined for granules or for branching hyphae in films stained on a slide.

6. **Immunology.** Agglutinins and complement-fixing antibodies can be demonstrated in individuals with the disease. However, at the present time methods are not sufficiently standardized for practical use.

7. **Special Requirements.** Species of *Actinomyces* are difficult to maintain in culture for stock supply. One of the best methods is lyophilization of a brain-heart infusion broth culture by taking the spun-down culture and sterilized milk, adding both to the lyophilization tubes, and lyophilizing the tubes. Pine and Watson (1959) have developed an *Actinomyces* maintenance medium. After the organism has grown in the liquid medium under pyrogallol-carbonate seal, the tube is kept in a deep freeze. If the tube is kept in the refrigerator, transfers should be made about every 6 months.

Questions:

1. List some similarities and differences between *Actinomyces* and *Nocardia*.

2. What are some differences between *Mycobacterium*, diptheroids, and *Actinomyces?*

3. In what ways do the Actinomycetes resemble the bacteria? The fungi?

4. How may *Actinomyces* and *Actinobacillus* be distinguished readily in the laboratory in pus taken from a cow with actinomycosis and a cow with actinobacillosis?

Selected References

1. AMAN, E. B. 1954. Actinomycosis (Actinomycosis in Animals). Southwest Veterin. 7:356.

2. AVERY, R. J. and F. Blank. 1954. On the chemical composition of cell walls of the Actinomycetales and its relation to their systematic position. Canad. J. Microbiol. 1:140.

3. BLANK, C. H. and L. K. Georg. 1968. The use of fluorescent antibody methods for the detection and identification of *Actinomyces species* in clinical material. J. Lab. Clin. Med. 71:283.

4. BOONE, C. J. and L. Pine. 1968. Rapid method for characterization of actinomycetes by cell wall composition. Appl. Microbiol. 16:279.

5. BROCK, D. W. and L. K. Georg. 1969. Determination and analysis of *Actinomyces israelii* serotypes 1 and 2. J. Bact. 97:581.

6. BROWN, J. M., L. K. Georg and L. C. Waters. 1969. Laboratory identification of *Rothia dentocariosa* and its occurrence in human clinical materials. Appl. Microbiol. 17:150.

7. COPE, V. Z. 1938. Actinomycosis. Oxford University Press, London.

8. CUMMINS, C. S. and H. Harris. 1958. Studies on the cell wall composition and taxonomy of Actinomycetales and related groups. J. Gen. Microbiol. 18:173.

9. EMMONS, C. W. 1938. The isolation of *Actinomyces bovis* from tonsilar granules. Pub. Health Rep. 53:1967.

10. ERIKSON, D. 1940. Pathogenic Anaerobic Organisms of the *Actinomyces* Group. Medical Research Council (Great Britain) Special Report Series No. 240.

11. ERIKSON, D. 1949. The morphology, cytology and taxonomy of the actinomycetes. Ann. Rev. Microbiol. 3:23.

12. FROST, B. M. 1940. A study of the *Actinomyces* in the mouths of normal cattle. Thesis, Cornell. Pp. 21.

13. GALE, D. and C. A. Waldron. 1955. Experimental actinomycosis with *Actinomyces israelii*. J. Infect. Dis. 97:251.

14. GEORG, L. K., G. W. Roberstad and S. A. Brinkman. 1964. Identification of species of *Actinomyces*. J. Bact. 88:477.

15. GEORG, L. K., G. W. Roberstad, S. A. Brinkman and M. D. Hicklin. 1965. A new pathogenic anaerobic *Actinomyces* species. J. Infect. Dis. 115.

16. GERENESER, M. A. and J. M. Slack. 1969. Identification of human strains of *Actinomyces viscosus*. Appl. Microbiol. 18:80.

17. HAZEN, E. L. and G. N. Little. 1958. *Actinomyces bovis* and "anaerobic diptheriods": Pathogenicity for hamsters and some other differentiating characteristics. J. Lab. Clin. Med. 51:968.

18. HOWELL, A., W. C. Murphy, F. Paul and R. M. Stephan. 1959. Oral strains of *Actinomyces*. J. Bact. 78:82.

19. KIMBALL, A., M. J. Tweihaus and E. R. Frank. 1954. *Actinomyces bovis* isolated from six cases of bovine orchitis. A preliminary report. Am. J. Vet. Res. 15:551.

20. KING, S. and E. Meyer. 1963. Gel diffusion technique in antigen-antibody reactions of *Actinomyces* species and "anaerobic diptheroids". J. Bact. 85:186.

21. LI, Y. -Y. F. and L. K. Georg. 1968. Differentiation of *Actinomyces propionicus* from *Actinomyces israelii* and *Actinomyces naeslundii* by gas chromatography. Can J. Microbiol. 14:749.

22. MENGES, R. W., H. W. Larsh and R. T. Habermann. 1953. Canine Actinomycosis. A report of two cases. J. Am. Vet. Med. Assoc. 122:73.

23. MEYER, E. and P. Verges. 1950. Mouse pathogenicity as a diagnostic aid in the identification of *Actinomyces bovis*. J. Lab. and Clin. Med. 36:667.

24. NEGRONI, P. and H. Bonfiglioli. 1939. *Actinomyces israelii* (Kruse). Physis. Rev. Soc. Argent. Ci. Nat. 15:151.

25. OLNEY, J. F. 1950. Actinomycosis - a new disease of turkeys. Vet. Med. 45:392.

26. PEABODY, J. W. and J. H. Seaburg. 1960. Actinomycosis and nocardiosis. A review of basic differences in therapy. Am. J. Med. 28:99.

27. PEGRUM, G. D. 1964. Actinomycotic lesions in the chorio-allantoic membrane of the chick embryo. J. Path. Bact. 88:323.

28. PINE, L., A. Howell and S. J. Watson. 1960. Studies on the morphological, physiological, and biochemical characteristics of *Actinomyces bovis*. J. Gen. Microbiol. 23:403.

29. PINE, L. and S. J. Watson. 1959. Evaluation of an isolation and maintenance medium for *Actinomyces* species and related organisms. J. Lab. and Clin. Med. 45:107.

30. PIRTLE, E. C. and P. A. Rebers and W. W. Weigel. 1965. Nitrogen-containing and carbohydrate-containing antigen from *Actinomyces bovis*. J. Bact. 89:880.

31. ROSEBURY, T., L. J. Epps and A. R. Clark. 1944. A study of the isolation, cultivation and pathogenicity of *Actinomyces israelii* recovered from the human mouth and from actinomycosis in man. J. Infect. Dis. 74:131.

32. RYFF, J. F. 1953. Encephalitis in a deer due to *Actinomyces bovis*. J. Am. Vet. Med. Assoc. 122:911.

33. SLACK, J. M. and N. A. Gerencser. 1966. Revision of serological grouping of *Actinomyces*. J. Bact. 91:2107.

34. SLACK, J. M., S. Landfried and M. A. Gerencser. 1969. Morphological, biochemical, and serological studies on 64 strains of *Actinomyces israelii*. J. Bact. 97:873.

35. SMITH, C. H. 1952. Ocular actinomycosis. Proc. Roy. Soc. Med. 46:209.

36. SOHLER, A., A. H. Romano and W. J. Nickerson. 1958. Biology of Actinomycetales. III. Cell wall composition. J. Bact. 75:283.

37. THOMPSON, L. 1950. Isolation and comparison of *Actinomyces* from human and bovine infections. Proc. Staff. Meet., Mayo Clinic 25:81.

38. WEED, L. A. and A. H. Baggenstoss. 1949. Actinomycosis: A pathologic and bacteriologic study of twenty-one fatal cases. Am. J. Clin. Path. 19:201.

NOCARDIOSIS

Definition:

Nocardiosis is an infection similar to actinomycosis in symptoms, with suppuration and granuloma in the subcutaneous tissues resulting in swelling, abscesses, and draining sinuses. The disease may be a primary pulmonary infection, later involving other organs, especially the brain and at times the kidneys, spleen, liver, and adrenals through hematogenous spread. Some species may develop mycetomas in the extremities (see mycetoma, p. 112). Note Plate XI.

Etiological Agents:

Nocardia asteroides (Eppinger) Blanchard, 1896, is the most common cause of nocardiosis throughout the world. A second agent, *N. brasiliensis* (Lindenberg) Castellani and Chalmers, 1913, may cause nocardiosis on occasions in the United States but is more common in Central and South America. Both organisms may also be the cause of mycetomas.

In addition to the two *Nocardia* species that may cause the actinomycotic mycetoma, there are several species of *Streptomyces*. In all cases the mycelial elements in the mycetoma are 1 μ or less in diameter in contrast to hyphae in the maduromycotic mycetoma granules. Species of *Streptomyces* causing mycetomas are: *Streptomyces madurae* (Vincent) Mackinnon and Artagaveytia-Allende, 1956 [*Nocardia madurae* (Vincent) Blanchard, 1896]; *Streptomyces pelletierii* (Lavern) Mackinnon and Artagaveytia-Allende, 1956; and *Streptomyces somaliensis* (Brumpt) Mackinnon and Artagaveytia-Allende, 1956. Note: On the basis of cell wall type, *S. madurae* should be *Nocardia madurae*, and *S. pelletierii* should be *N. pelletierii*.

Nocardia farcinica, as considered by Trevisan, infects cattle, causing tumefactions and granulomatous inflammation, lymph node involvement, and subcutaneous tissues. The morphology and biochemical reactions are similar to *N. asteroides*. Gordon and Mihm (1962) suggested that *N. farcinica* be reduced to synonomy with *N. asteroides*. The status of this species is in doubt.

Occurrence:

Nocardia asteroides has been isolated from soil a number of times and once from skin on a foot. Gonzales-Ochoa (1961) reported *N. brasiliensis* from a soil sample in Mexico. The infection is exogenous, introduced through injury, or following inhalation of the fungus.

1. **Man:** Nocardiosis due to *N. asteroides* occurs throughout the world, while the disease due to *N. brasiliensis* has been reported in Mexico, Central America, South America, North America, India, and Africa.

   The actinomycotic mycetomas occur more frequently in the subtropics and tropics. These areas include Africa, South America, Mexico, India, Europe, and Australia. *Streptomyces somaliensis* is more common in Africa, *S. pelletierii* is more likely in Africa and South America, while *S. madurae* is worldwide in distribution, including the United States.

2. **Animals:** A number of infections due to *N. asteroides* have been reported in dogs, cows, and rainbow trout (Snieszko et al., 1964). For reference to other species see *Fungal Diseases of Animals* by Ainsworth and Austwick (1959).

Laboratory Procedures

1. **Source of Infected Material:** Pus, sputum, or tissue should be collected in a sterile container. Cerebrospinal fluid should be brought in the laboratory in the same manner for centrifugation to concentrate sediment for examination. Biopsy or autopsy specimens may be available for laboratory study. Usually granules are not present in the infected material in nocardiosis cases, but would be in mycetoma cases.

2. **Examination of Infected Material:**

   a. Prepare smears of pus, sputum, or centrifuged sediment, and stain with Gram and the modified Kinyoun acid-fast stain for examination. The decolorization with acid alcohol should not exceed 5 to 10 seconds.

   b. Microscopically, the smears are always Gram-positive with branching hyphae 1 μ in diameter, or bacillary and coccoid forms (Plate XXI). The results of the acid-fast stain will vary according to species.

3. **Cultures:** Infected materials will grow on Sabouraud glucose agar without antibiotics. The species of *Nocardia* are sensitive to antibacterial antibiotics. Digestion of contaminated material may increase the chance for isolation of *N. asteroides* by reducing competition of contaminating microorganisms. Cultures should be incubated at 25° and 37° C. Species are separated on the basis of pigmentation, colony characteristic, morphology, acid-fastness, hydrolysis of casein, amylolytic activity, and other biochemical reactions (Table VII). Hyphae of these species are less than 1 μ in diameter. Isolation by paraffin bait technique is useful (p. 41).

   In the laboratory studies compare *N. asteroides* with *N. brasiliensis*. Stain slides with Gram and acid-fast stains to check microscopic appearance. Compare cultural and biochemical characteristics for both species. The following two species are etiological agents of nocardiosis. The last three are causes of actinomycotic mycetomas (see maduromycosis).

   a. *Nocardia asteroides:* On Sabouraud glucose agar, the colonies are fast-growing, glabrous, chalky, folded or wrinkled, white to orange-pink in color, and have aerial hyphae. On Czapek agar the color is yellow to orange (see Plate XXI). 37° C. optimum. Grows at 46° C.

      Microscopically, smears show Gram-positive, branched hyphae fragmenting into bacillary forms. Partially, or acid-fast (see Plate XXI). Chains of conidia may form.

   b. *N. brasiliensis:* On Sabouraud agar, the colonies are fast-growing, folded, cerebriform, white to orange in color, dry and chalky, or glabrous with an earthy odor. On Czapek agar the colonies are similar in appearance. 30° C. optimum. Terminal conidia may be present. Does not grow at 46° C.

      Microscopically, stained slides are Gram-positive with mycelium fragmenting into different length bacillary forms. Partially, or acid-fast. Similar to *N. asteroides.*

AGENTS OF ACTINOMYCOTIC MYCETOMA

   a. *S. madurae:* The colonies on Sabouraud agar are glabrous, waxy, wrinkled, moist, granular, cream to occasionally red in color (Plate XXI). On Czapek agar the colonies are cream colored at first, and later pink to red in color. 37° C. optimum.

      Microscopically, smears are Gram-positive, with delicate hyphae that do not fragment. Chains of spherical condia may be formed in some isolates. Not acid fast (see Plate XXI).

   b. *S. pelletierii:* On Sabouraud agar colonies develop slowly with a wrinkled, heaped, glabrous surface and a coral pink to red color. On Czapek agar the colonies are coral red. 37° C. optimum.

      Microscopically, stained slides are Gram-positive with delicate, branched hyphae that do not fragment. Not acid-fast.

   c. *S. somaliensis:* The colonies grow slowly with a creamy, wrinkled or folded, leathery surface. A white to tan aerial hyphal growth may develop. Older colonies may become dark gray to brown. 30° C. optimum.

      Microscopically, stained slides have nonfragmenting, delicate branched hyphae. Conidia may be present. Not acid-fast.

Nocardiosis

COLONY

ORGANISMS IN CULTURE

ORGANISM IN TISSUE

145 Nocardia asteroides

146 Hyphae-Acid Fast stain

147 Organism in pus

148 Streptomyces madurae

149 S. madurae hyphae-acid fast stain

150 Nocardia brasiliensis

PLATE XXI

TABLE VII
Characteristics of Species of *Nocardia* and *Streptomyces*

Species	Granule	Fragmentation hyphae	Acid-fast	Cell wall type*	Casein hydrolysis	Decomposition of tyrosine	Decomposition of xanthine	Amylolytic activity	Utilization of paraffin	Liquefy gelatin	Urease
N. asteroides	white to yellow if present, about 1 mm; absent if systemic.	+	+	IV	−	−	−	−	+	−	+
N. brasiliensis	Like above, granules more common, with or without clubs.	+	+	IV	+	+	−	−	+	+	+
S. madurae (N. madurae)	White to yellow or red, large, 1-10 mm, soft, lobulated.	−	−	III	+	+ *(− for 14%)**	−	+	−	+	−
S. pelletierii (N. pelletierii)	red, smooth-edged, hard, 0.3-0.5 mm.	−	−	III	+	+	−	− *(+ for 13%)**	−	+	−
S. somaliensis	Yellow to brown, hard, 1-2 mm, round.	−	−	I	+	+	−	±	−	+	−
Streptomyces sp. *(saprophytes)*	− −	−	Spores usually +	I	+ (or) −	+	− (or) +	+ (usual)	− (usual)	+ (usual)	±

*Cell walls of actinomycetes have glucoasmine, muramic acid, glutamic acid, and alanine. Individual groups contain the following components: (I) LL-diaminopimelic acid (DAP) and glycine; (III) meso-DAP; (IV) meso-DAP, arabinose, and galactose (Becker, 1965).

** Gordon (1966).

TECHNIQUES FOR NOCARDIA AND
STREPTOMYCES IDENTIFICATION

a. <u>Stains</u>. For procedure and preparation of stains for Gram and acid-fast stains (Kinyoun's modification) see Staining Methods, pages 32-33.

b. <u>Casein Medium</u>. For preparation of this medium to check proteolytic activity, see Media for Specific Use, page 41. Streak or make single point inoculations of each organism on the plates, and at the end of 1 and 2 weeks check for clearing of casein. *N. asteroides* will not hydrolyze casein.

c. <u>Gelatin Liquefaction</u>. Check the gelatin liquefaction reaction on the nutrient broth gelatin medium (see page 41 for preparation). Inoculate the organisms slightly below the surface of the medium and incubate either at 24° or 37° C, along with a control. After growth occurs, refrigerate until control solidifies and check for liquefaction.

d. <u>Other biochemical tests.</u> Organisms should be inoculated into tyrosine (see page 42) and xanthine and starch-agar plates for characteristic species reactions. Urease test broth should be used to determine the reaction for urease. Utilization of paraffin may readily be determined.

4. **Histopathology.** If biopsy or autopsy material is available, sections should be made and stained by Gram stain to demonstrate branching hyphae or the granules if present. The hyphae are also readily shown by the Gomori-methenamine silver stain. Periodic acid-Schiff stain is not satisfactory, nor is H and E stain, for demonstrating nocardiosis. A suppurative tissue reaction is usually evident in most cases. The separate hyphae or granules containing hyphae usually are found in the abscesses. For additional information see references.

5. **Animal Inoculation:** For routine diagnostic work, it is not necessary to check animal pathogenicity as identification is based on morphology and biochemical activity. The virulence among strains varies considerably, making it necessary to select strains and inoculate larger numbers of animals for demonstration of pathogenicity. The use of 5% gastric mucin is of value in increasing the susceptibility of the animal. The guinea pig, rabbit, and mouse have been reported to be susceptible to experimental nocardiosis.

Pathogenicity test for *Nocardia* species (Georg et al., 1961): After a heavy colony growth has developed on several tubes of Sabouraud glucose agar (about 1 to 2 weeks), scrape the growth from the slant into a mortar, and add an equal amount of 5% gastric mucin before grinding. Inject 1 ml intraperitoneally into at least 2 guinea pigs. If the animal dies or at the end of 2 and 4 weeks, autopsy the animals and examine for the presence of lesions with acid-fast hyphae.

Male mice may be inoculated intravenously with 0.2 ml of a 0.1% suspension of the pathogenic species of *Nocardia* and at the same time a 0.5 ml amount of a 5% gastric mucin suspension injected intraperitoneally. In 2 weeks the organism should be isolated from the spleen if it is pathogenic (Mohapatra and Pine, 1963). Both *N. asteroides* and *N. brasiliensis* can maintain viability in tissues for up to 3 weeks.

6. **Special tests for Presumptive identification.** Gordon and Mihm (1962) have suggested a presumptive identification of several *Nocardia* species as follows: An actinomycete with aerial hyphae that does not utilize casein, L-tyrosine, or xanthine may tentatively be considered *N. asteroides*. If a similar organism is acid-fast, utilizes casein and tyrosine, but not xanthine, it should be *N. brasiliensis*. Similar forms that decompose xanthine, but not casein or tyrosine may be considered *N. caviae*. Acid-fastness may vary in all three.

<u>Questions</u>:

1. What are the characteristics used to separate species of *Nocardia?*

2. Compare *Nocardia* with *Actinomyces* and *Streptomyces*.

3. What other fungi may cause mycetomas (maduromycosis)?

Selected References

1. AL DOORY, Y. 1965. Fluorescent antibody studies with *Nocardia asteroides*. Sabouraudia 4:135.

2. AINSWORTH, G. C. and P. K. C. Austwick. 1959. Fungal Diseases of Animals. Commonwealth Agricultural Bureaux. Franham Royal Bucks. England.

3. BECKER, B., M. P. Lechevalier and H. A. Lechevalier. 1965. Chemical composition of cell-wall preparations from strains of various form-genera of aerobic actinomycetes. Appl. Microbiol. 13:236.

4. BISHOP, C. T. and F. Blank. 1958. The chemical composition of Actinomycetales: Isolation of a polysaccharide containing arabinose and d-galactose from *Nocardia asteroides*. Canad. J. Microbiol. 4:35.

5. BLAKE, W. P. 1954. A report of two canine cases of nocardiosis in Missouri. J. Am. Vet. Med. Assoc. 125:467.

6. BOJALIL, L. F. and J. Cerbon. 1959. Scheme for the differentiation of *Nocardia asteroides* and *Nocardia brasiliensis*. J. Bact. 78:852.

7. CALERO, C. 1947. Madura foot (mycetoma). Arch. Derm. and Syph. 55:761.

8. FARSTCHI, D. 1967. Studies of the lipids of *Nocardia asteroides* isolates. Diss. Abstr. 28(6) B:2252. University of Georgia.

9. FAWI, M. F. 1964. Complement fixing antibodies in nocardiosis with special reference to dogs. Sabouraudia 3:303.

10. FREESE, J. W., W. G. Young, W. C. Sealy and N. F. Conant. 1963. Pulmonary infection by *Nocardia asteroides*. Findings in eleven clinical cases. J. Thorac. Cardiov. Surg. 46:537.

11. GEORG, L. K., L. Ajello, C. McDurmont and T. S. Hosty. 1961. The identification of *Nocardia asteroides* and *Nocardia brasiliensis*. Am. Rev. Respir. Dis. 84:337.

12. GONZALES-MENDOZA, A. and F. Mariat. 1964. Sur L'hydrolyze da la Gelatine comme caractere differentiel entre *Nocardia asteroides* et *N. brasiliensis*. Ann. Inst. Pasteur (Paris) 107: 560.

13. GORDON, R. E. and M. M. Smith. 1955. Proposed group of characters for the separation of *Streptomyces* and *Nocardia*. J. Bact. 67:147.

14. GORDON, R. E. and J. M. Mihm. 1962. Identification of *Nocardia caviae* (Erickson) *Nov.* comb. Ann. N. Y. Acad. Sci. 98:628.

15. GORDON, R. E. 1966. Some criteria for the recognition of *Nocardia madurae* (Vincent) Blanchard. J. Gen. Microbiol. 45:355.

16. HENDERSON, J. W., W. E. Wellman and L. A. Weed. 1960. Nocardiosis of the eye: Report of a case. Staff Meeting Mayo Clinic 35:614.

17. HOSTY, T. S., C. McDurmont, L. Ajello, L. K. Georg, G. L. Brumfield and A. A. Calix. 1961. Prevalence of *Nocardia asteroides* in sputa examined by a tuberculosis diagnostic laboratory. J. Lab. Clin. Med. 58:107.

18. HUPPERT, M., L. G. Wayne and W. J. Juarez. 1957. Characterization of atypical Mycobacteria and *Nocardia* species isolated from clinical specimens. II. Procedures for differentiating between acid-fast microorganisms. Am. Rev. Tb. Pul. Dis. 76:468.

19. KINGSBURY, E. W. and J. M. Slack. 1969. A polypeptide skin test antigen from *Nocardia asteroides*. II. Further studies on the specificity of a Nocardin active polypeptide. Sabouraudia 7:85.

20. KURUP, P. V., H. S. Randhawa and R. S. Sandhu. 1968. A survey of *Nocardia asteroides, N. caviae* and *N. brasiliensis* occurring in soil in India. Sabouraudia 6:260.

21. KWAPINSKI, J. B. and H. P. R. Seeliger. 1965. Investigations on the antigenic structure of Actinomycetales. IX. Serological classification of the Nocardiae with the polysaccharide fractions of their cell walls. Mycopathologia 25:173.

22. MACKINNON, J. E. and R. C. Artagaveytia-Allende. 1956. The main species of pathogenic aerobic Actinomycetes causing mycetomas. Roy. Soc. Trop. Med. Hyg. 50:31.

23. MARIAT, F. 1954. Physiologie des actinomycètes aérobies pathogènes. I. Expériences préliminaires. Ann. Inst. Pasteur 86:479.

24. Mc CLUNG, N. M. 1961. Isolation of *Nocardia asteroides* from soils. Mycologia 52:154.

25. Mc CLUNG, N. M. and I. Uesaka. 1961. Morphological studies in the genus *Nocardia*. VI. Aerial hyphal production and acid-fastness of *N. asteroides* isolates. Rev. Latinoamer. Microbiol. 4:97.

26. MOHAPATRA, L. N. and L. Pine. 1963. Studies on the pathogenicity of aerobic actinomycetes inoculated into mice intravenously. Sabouraudia 2:176.

27. MOSTAFA, I. E., L. Cerny and J. Cerna. 1968. Canine nocardiosis due to *Nocardia caviae*. Revue Élev. Méd. Vét. Pays Trop. 21:181.

28. PEABODY, J. W. and J. H. Seabury. 1960. Actinomycosis and nocardiosis. A review of basic differences in therapy. Am. J. Med. 28:99.

29. PIER, A. C., D. M. Gray and M. J. Fossatti. 1958. *Nocardia asteroides,* a newly recognized pathogen of the mastitis complex. Am. J. Vet. Res. 19:319.

30. PIER, A. C. and R. F. Keeler. 1965. Extracellular antigens of *Nocardia asteroides*. I. Production and immunologic characterization. Am. Rev. Resp. Dis. 91:391.

31. RIPPON, J. W. 1968. Extracellular collagenase produced by *Streptomyces madurae*. Biochim. Biophys. Acta. 159:147.

32. RIPPON, J. W. and G. Peck. 1967. Experimental infection with *Streptomyces (Nocardia) madurae*. J. Invest. Derm. 49:371.

33. SALTZMAN, H. A., E. W. Chick and N. F. Conant. 1962. Nocardiosis as a complication of other diseases. Lab. Invest. 11:1110.

34. SNIESZKO, S. F., G. L. Bullock, C. E. Dunbar and L. L. Pettijohn. 1964. Nocardial infection in hatchery-reared fingerling rainbow trout (*Salmo gairdneri*) J. Bact. 88:1809.

35. STROPNIK, Z. 1965. Isolation of *Nocardia asteroides* from human skin. Sabouraudia 4:41.

STREPTOTRICHOSIS

(Mycotic Dermatitis, Dermatophilosis)

Definition:

Streptotrichosis is an exudative pustular dermatitis of the skin followed by the formation of scabs and crusts. Alopecia may be evident after scabs and crusts fall off in healed areas.

Etiological Agent:

Dermatophilus congolensis Van Saceghem 1915. Isolates from cattle, sheep, horses, and deer have been assigned other names. Gordon (1964) considers these variations of *D. congolensis.*

Occurrence:

1. **Man:** The organism has been reported in humans living in the United States: in Texas, Iowa, and New York.

2. **Animals:** This disease is frequently found in cattle, sheep, and at times in goats, horses, other domestic animals, and feral mammals. The disease in cattle is commonly known as "mycotic dermatitis," in sheep as "lumpy wool" or "strawberry foot rot."

Laboratory Procedures

1. **Source of Infected Material:** Crusts and scabs from the animal placed in containers should be brought into the laboratory for examination and for culture.

2. **Examination of Infected Material:**

   a. Smears may be prepared from the scabs or crusts and suspended in saline. Giemsa or methylene blue are good to stain the smear. For tissue sections, Hematoxylin and Eosin, Giemsa, or Grocott silver stain may be used (Gordon, 1970).

   b. <u>Microscopically</u>, the organism may be seen in any of the various stages of its life cycle in the cellular serous exudate or keratinizing cells of the superficial epithelia or hair follicle epithelia. The characteristic branched filaments divide both transversely and longitudinally to develop packets of coccoid forms. The branched filaments are 2 to 5 μ in diameter. Motility is usually evident, and clusters of spores may be germinating.

3. **Cultures:** The organism may be isolated in pure culture by streaking the exudate (taken from a closed pustule) on blood agar plates. If the crust or scab is contaminated, immerse in a bottle of distilled water for 3¼ hours at 24° C., expose to CO_2 in a candle jar for 15 minutes, and streak the surface film of the water containing the zoospores onto the agar medium (Haalstra, 1965).

   a. <u>Dermatophilus congolensis.</u> On blood agar at 37° C. the colonies develop in 24 hours as small round, square or irregular, grayish-white, raised rough, hard, adherent and usually form pits in the medium. In 2 to 5 days an orange pigment usually develops. Betahemolysis develops on beef heart infusion-horse blood agar. Colonies vary from white to orange, and may be granular or membranous on brain-heart infusion slants at 37° C, depending on the strain. In beef infusion-peptone broth at 37° C there is a thick sediment while the supernatant fluid is clear.

   b. <u>Microscopically</u>, in wet, unstained mounts or with methylene blue stain, look for branched filaments, segmentation stage, cocci arranged irregularly in cube-shaped packets or the clusters of germinating spores. Check for motility of coccoid spores, about 0.5 to 1.0 μ in diameter.

4. **Biochemical Reactions:** The organism is catalase positive, and the urease test is positive. Casein and starch are decomposed while xanthine is not. Gelatin is liquefied and nitrates are reduced while indole is not produced.

5. **Laboratory Animals:** These are not necessary for identification of *D. congolensis,* but may be helpful in detecting and isolating the organism from specimens brought in for isolation in the laboratory. The abraded skin of a rabbit, guinea pig, or mouse is inoculated with the organism. Acute ulcerative pustular dermatitis mostly around the hair follicles should develop.

Questions:

1. Compare *Dermatophilus* with *Nocardia* microscopically, in culture, and in the tissue of the patient.

Selected References

1. DEAN, D. J., M. A. Gordon, C. W. Severinghaus, E. T. Kroll and J. R. Reilly. 1961. Streptothricosis: A new zoonotic disease. N. Y. State J. Med. 61:1283.
2. GORDON, M. A. 1964. The genus *Dermatophilus.* J. Bacteriol. 88:509.
3. GORDON, M. A. 1970. Chapter 15 in *Manual of Clinical Microbiology.* Ed. by J. E. Blair, E. H. Lennette, and J. P. Truant. Published by American Society for Microbiology. Bethesda, Md.
4. HAALSTRA, R. T. 1965. Isolation of *Dermatophilus congolensis* from skin lesions in the diagnosis of streptothricosis. Vet. Rec. 77:824.
5. KAPLAN, W. 1966. Dermatophilosis — a recently recognized disease in the United States. S. West Vet. 20:140.
6. LE RICHE, P. D. 1968. The transmission of dermatophilosis in sheep. Aust. Vet. J. 44:64.
7. LEUDEMANN, G. M. 1968. *Geodermatophilus,* a new genus of the Dermatophilaceae (Actinomycetales). J. Bact. 96:1848.
8. ROBERTS, D. S. 1965. Cutaneous actinomycosis due to the single species *Dermatophilus congolensis.* Nature 206:1068.
9. ROBERTS, D. S. 1967. *Dermatophilus* infection. Vet. Bull. 37:513.
10. SERCY, G. P. and T. J. Hulland. *Dermatophilus dermatitis* (streptotrichosis) in Ontario. I. Clinical observations. II. Laboratory findings. Can. Vet. J. 9:7.

MISCELLANEOUS MYCOSES

This group of unrelated fungus diseases are less frequently encountered. Some of these diseases may be occurring more frequently in recent years as a result of opportunistic conditions for development when patients have been receiving antimicrobial and steroid drugs for treatment of other diseases. In addition to rhinosporidiosis, phycomycosis, cladosporiosis, and aspergillosis, there are occasionally a few others including penicilliosis. Reference should be made to aspergillosis following the colored PLATE XVII.

Many of these fungi are usually considered saprophytes when isolated from lesions or internally. If a fungus is isolated more than once and in quantity from a lesion or sputum, and other etiological agents are ruled out, then this isolate is significant and may be the causative agent of the disease. An isolate from an internal organ, from an enclosed body cavity, or on blood culture should be considered of greater possible significance.

RHINOSPORIDIOSIS

Definition:

Rhinosporidiosis is a chronic granulomatous infection of polypoid tumors or pedunculated and sessile polyps in the mucous membranes of the nose, eyes, ears, larynx, and rarely on other parts of the body.

Etiological Agent:

The disease is caused by *Rhinosporidium seeberi* (Wernicke) Seeber, 1912.

Occurrence:

1. **Man:** The fungus, although difficult to culture, apparently is found in water or possibly as a fish disease. Rhinosporidiosis is found more often in India and in Ceylon, as well as Brazil, with occasional reports in the United States, Mexico, Cuba, Argentina, Ecuador, Paraguay, Russia, Iran, Africa, the Philippines, the Malay States, Italy, England, and Scotland. Over 1000 cases have occurred in India and Ceylon, and more than 200 have been reported in Brazil.

2. **Animals:** The disease has been found in horses, mules, cattle, and dogs, especially in India, South America, South Africa, Australia, and the United States.

Laboratory Procedures

1. **Source of Infected Material:** Material from the polyps that have been removed surgically should be brought to the laboratory under sterile conditions for examination.

2. **Examination of Infected Material:**

   a. The exudate of the material may be examined directly (or sectioned for better results) by squeezing gently and placing in water on a slide, adding a cover glass on top, and making a microscopic examination. In addition, smears may be made with the exudate or nasal secretions and stained.

   b. <u>Microscopically</u>, the direct slide mount or stained tissue sections, if positive, should show round or oval spores, 7-9 μ in diameter, as well as sporangia filled with spores (Fig. 53, Plate XXII). The life cycle, as described by Ashworth (1923) and others, consists of:

      (1) The round, thickened-chitinous wall spore, 6-7 μ in diameter, contains a nucleus with four chromosomes.

      (2) The infecting spore enlarges up to 50 or 60 μ in diameter along with many nuclear divisions.

      (3) Further nuclear divisions and enlargement occurs until the cell is 100 μ in diameter. A thick layer of cellulose is deposited inside the chitinous membrane except at one point where a pore begins to appear.

      (4) Further nuclear divisions occur with cleavage and rounding up of the cytoplasm which eventually result in a sporangium with nearly 4000 protoplasmic units.

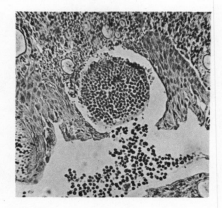

Figure 53
Sporangium with spores

(5) Two more nuclear divisions result in approximately 16,000 spores, 7-9 μ in diameter at maturity in an enlarged (spherule) sporangium up to 300 μ in diameter.

3. **Cultures**: Grover (1970) has attempted to study the organism in culture in a liquid medium (developed by Morgan, Campbell and Morton, 1955).

4. **Pathological Studies**: If prepared, stained slides are available for demonstration, study the stages in the life cycle of the fungus and pathological changes. Note that ruptured sporangia may be seen. Released spores from the sporangia incite a polymorphonuclear inflammatory reaction and abscess formation. Further changes commonly show a chronic type inflammation with plasma cells and lymphocytes most conspicuous. For further details, see reference books.

5. **Animal Inoculation**: There are no reports of successful infection of laboratory animals.

Questions:

1. Diagram the life cycle of the organism.

2. Compare and contrast the tissue phase of *Rhinosporidium seeberi* with *Coccidioides immitis*. Are there any differences in location of the infection and laboratory procedures for identification?

Selected References

1. ASHWORTH, J. H. 1923. On *Rhinosporidium seeberi* (Wernicke, 1903) with special reference to its sporulation and affinities. Trans. Roy. Soc. Edinb. 53(2):301.
2. CALDWELL, G. T. and J. D. Roberts. 1938. Rhinosporidiosis in the United States. J. Am. Med. Assoc. 110-1641.
3. CHRISTIAN, E. C. and J. Kovi. 1966. Three cases of rhinosporidiosis in Ghana. Ghana Med. J. 5:63.
4. DUBE, B. and G. D. Veliath. 1964. Rhinosporidiosis in Mangalore. J. Indian Med. Assoc. 42:59.
5. GROVER, S. 1970. *Rhinosporidium seeberi;* a preliminary study of the morphology and life cycle. Sabouraudia 7:249.
6. KAMESWARAN, S. 1966. Surgery in rhinosporidiosis. Experience with 293 cases. Int. Surg. 46:602.
7. KARPOVA, M. F. 1964. On the morphology of rhinosporidiosis. Mycopathologia 23:281.
8. KARUNARATNE, W. A. E. 1964. Rhinosporidiosis in Man. x/146 pp. 1 col. pl, 28 pl. The Athlone Press, London.
9. KURIAKOSE, E. T. 1963. Oculosporidiosis. Rhinosporidiosis of the eye. Br. J. Ophthal. 47: 346.
10. MORGAN, J. F., M. E. Campbell and H. J. Morton. 1955. Nutrition of animal tissues cultivated in vitro. Survey of natural materials as supplements to synthetic medium. J. Nat. Cancer. Inst. 16:557.
11. MYERS, D. D., J. Simon and M. T. Case. 1964. Rhinosporidiosis in a horse. J. Am. Vet. Med. Assoc. 145:345.
12. NINO, F. L. and R. S. Freire. 1966. Existensia de un foco endemico de rinosporidiosis en la provincia del Chaco. Nuevas observaciones de r. equina. Caracteres ecologicos de la region de Villa Angela. Revta Med. Vet., B. Aires. 47:521.
13. VEGA-NÚÑEZ, J. and D. A. Herrero. 1966. Dos casos de rinosporidiosis familiar. Dermatologia, Méx. 10:498.

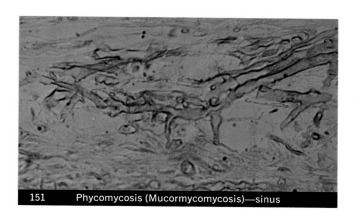

151   Phycomycosis (Mucormycomycosis)—sinus

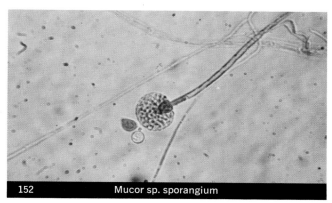

152   Mucor sp. sporangium

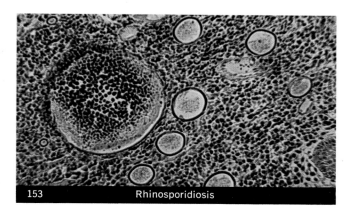

153   Rhinosporidiosis

Plate XXII

PHYCOMYCOSIS

(Mucormycosis)

Definition:

Phycomycosis is a disease caused by fungi in the class Phycomycetes. The disease may be rapidly fatal unless specific treatment diverts the course of the infection. Phycomycosis may occur in the central nervous system, cornea, subcutaneous tissue, lungs, and gastrointestinal tract. The fungi may invade when resistance is low through the mucous membrane, through the lung, or they may penetrate the lumen of the blood vessels to produce acute inflammation and vascular thrombosis and may reach the central nervous system to produce a meningo-encephalitis.

Etiological Agents:

Various species of *Mucor, Rhizopus, Absidia, Mortierella, Basidiobolus* and *Entomophthora* may be pathogenic. *Entomophthora* sp. and *Hyphomyces destruens* have been reported as causative agents in animals.

Occurrence:

The disease usually occurs in individuals with metabolic disturbances such as cases where diabetes was not controlled or malnutrition and other conditions are associated as acidosis. Other predisposing factors include increased use of corticosteroides, antibiotics, and antileukemic drugs.

1. **Man:** The disease is worldwide in distribution. The organisms are common in decaying vegetation as saprophytes and laboratory contaminants, becoming pathogens under certain conditions as indicated. A subcutaneous phycomycosis caused by *Basidiobolus meristosporus* occurs in Asia and Africa.

2. **Animals:** The disease has been reported in dogs, birds, horses, sheep, cows, pigs, mink, guinea pigs, and mice.

Laboratory Procedures

1. **Source of Infected Material:** There is considerable difficulty in obtaining material in most cases, except after biopsy, autopsy, or from slides made for pathological study. In case of central nervous system phycomycosis, material should be taken from the nasal mucosa and from the sinuses for direct mounts. Scrapings or biopsy should be made for cutaneous type infections. Abscesses should be aspirated.

2. **Examination of Infected Material:** Direct KOH examination on slide mounts of sputum or scraped material should show nonseptate mycelium and rounded sporangia if present. Stained sections on slides made from pathological tissue will show the same structures as in direct examination of material (Fig. 54). The hyphae are nonseptate and 6-50 μ in width.

3. **Cultures:** All of the organisms grow on Sabouraud glucose agar with or without the addition of antibacterial antibiotics. Cycloheximide should not be used in the medium for isolation of any of the Phycomycetes. All are fast-growing, usually spreading over a plate in a few days, with an abundance of aerial mycelium. Incubate at 25° C and 37° C.

   NOTE: Since all genera except *Basidiobolus* and *Entomophthora* are common laboratory contaminants, the isolation of these genera in culture becomes significant if nonseptate hyphae are found in the specimen taken from the patient. Repeated isolation of the same organism from the patient is of value.

a. *Rhizopus* sp.

Growth is rapid, filling the plate with a cottony surface in a few days. See contaminants for additional information on the colony and microscopic appearance of *Rhizopus* sp. All species usually produce sporangiophores that arise directly from a cluster of rhizoids.

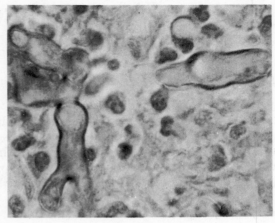

Figure 54
Mucor sp. in Tissue, x 1200.

(1) *R. oryzae* Went and Prinsen-Geerlings, 1895 is the most frequently reported isolate from phycomycosis.

Colony: The fast-growing white colonies become yellowish-brown in color with dark-brown sporangia soon appearing.

Microscopically, the nonseptate hyphae have very long sporangiophores (up to 200 μ) with yellowish-brown rhizoids. The sporangia form light-brown, striated, irregularly formed spores, 6-8 by 5-6 μ in size. Zygospores not known.

(2) *R. arrhizus* Fischer, 1892 is like *R. stolonifer (R. nigricans)* except spores are about one-half as large or 5-7 μ in diameter, and the rhizoids are not as well-developed.

(3) *R. stolonifer* (Ehrenberg ex Fries) Viuill. *(R. nigricans)* has spores 7-15 μ in diameter, and the rhizoids are well developed.

b. *Absidia* sp. The species usually reported in phycomycosis is *A. corymbifera* (Cohn) Saccardo and Trotter, 1912.

Colony: The growth of the fungus gives a course gray, woolly appearance. The rate of growth is about the same as for *Rhizopus*.

Microscopically, the sporangiophores are formed between nodes on the internodes of the stolon instead of the nodes as in *Rhizopus*. The sporangia are somewhat pear-shaped with a columella in each. The spores are round to oval, 2-3 by 3-4 μ in size.

c. *Mucor* sp.

Colony: Species of *Mucor* grow rapidly, forming a cottony surface that may partially fill a petri dish or completely fill it. The mycelium is white at first, becoming gray to yellowish-brown.

Microscopically, the nonseptate hyphae have no rhizoid formation. Sporangiophores arise from the hyphae, forming terminal sporangia with columellae. The sporangiophores may be branched. Zygospores may be formed by some species. There is considerable variation in sporangia, spore size, and color in different species of *Mucor*.

d. *Mortierella* sp.

Colony: Most isolated from human cases have little aerial hyphae produced on the surface of the gray or yellowish colony.

Microscopically, the sporangiophores usually taper to a narrow tip where the sporangium is attached. Branches may occur on the sporangiophores. The sporangium has no columella and small spores about 1-2 by 2-4 μ. Smaller, one-celled conidia or "stylospores" that are spiny or echinulate may be present.

e. *Basidiobolus ranarum* Eidam 1887.

Colony: The organism grows as a thin, glabrous, flat colony on the surface of Sabouraud agar with a gray to yellow color.

Microscopically, the hyphae form numerous club-shaped sporangiophores with a pear-shaped sporangium that is discharged by force. Later this uninucleate sporangium divides and forms spores inside. Two adjacent cells may unite to form rough, thick-walled zygospores. Later thick-walled chlamydospores may be the only special structures formed by the hyphae.

4. **Histopathology**: The hyphae causing phycomycosis stain well with H and E. Stains such as Gridley and PAS are not satisfactory. The hyphae are usually present in abundance in infected tissues where there is extensive polymorphonuclear infiltration and necrosis. The hyphae tend to be around the blood vessels as well as show infiltration of the walls. The hyphae are non-septate and wider than *Aspergillus,* or around 15-20 μ in diameter, and up to 200 μ in length.

5. **Animal Inoculation**: Cerebral and pulmonary mucormycosis has been reported in rabbits (made diabetic with alloxan and injecting the rabbit with either *R. oryzae* or *R. arrhizus;* Baker, 1955). Mice inoculated intraperitoneally with 1 ml. of 10% suspension of ground *R. arrhizus* may develop inflammatory masses with hyphae in the peritoneum. Masses should be found in the upper quadrant binding the liver, spleen, pancreas, and stomach together. The animals recover in about 4 weeks. Animals are not sufficiently susceptible to be useful in determining pathogenicity.

Questions:

1. What are the predisposing factors that aid in the development of phycomycosis?

2. How does the tissue phase of phycomycosis differ from aspergillosis?

3. What are differences and similarities between *Rhizopus, Mucor, Mortierella* and *Absidia?*

4. What is the difference between causative agents of subcutaneous phycomycosis and phycomycosis, and the development of the two diseases?

Selected References

1. BAKER, R. D. 1957. Mucormycosis — A new disease? J. Am. Med. Assoc. 163:805.
2. BATTOCK, D. J., H. Grausz, M. Bobrowsky and M. L. Littman. 1968. Alternate-day amphotericin B therapy in the treatment of rhinocerebral phycomycosis (mucormycosis). Ann. Intern. Med. 68:122.
3. BAUER, H., L. Ajello, E. Adams and D. U. Hernandez. 1955. Cerebral Mucormycosis; Pathogenesis of the disease. Am. J. Med. 18:822.
4. BAUER, H., G. L. Wallace, Jr. and W. H. Sheldon. 1957. The effects of cortisone and chemical inflammation on experimental mucormycosis (*Rhizopus oryzae* infections). Yale J. Biol. & Med. 29:389.
5. COCKSHOTT, W. P., B. M. Clark and F. D. Martinson. 1968. Upper respiratory infection due to *Entomophthora coronata.* Radiology 90:1016.
6. CORDES, D. O., W. A. Royal and E. H. Shortridge. 1967. Systemic mycosis in neonatal calves. N. Z. Vet. J. 15:143.
7. DAVIS, C. L., W. A. Anderson and B. R. McCrory. 1955. Mucormycosis in food-producing animals. A report of 12 cases. J. Am. Vet. Med. Assoc. 126:261.
8. EMMONS, C. W. 1964. Phycomycosis in Man and Animals. Riv. Pat. veg., Pavia, Ser. 3, 4:329.
9. GINSBERG, J., A. G. Spaulding and V. O. Laing. 1966. Cerebral phycomycosis (mucormycosis) with ocular involvement. Am. J. Ophthal. 62:900.
10. GREER, D. L. and L. Friedman. 1964. Effect of temperature on growth as a differentiating characteristic between human and nonhuman isolates of *Basidiobolus* species. J. Bact. 88:812.
11. GREER, D. L. and L. Friedman. 1966. Studies on the genus *Basidiobolus* with reclassification of the species pathogenic for man. Sabouraudia 4:231.
12. GRUEBER, H. L. E. 1969. Rhino-entomophthoromycosis. J. Christian Med. Ass. India 44:20.

13. HARRIS, J. S. 1955. Mucormycosis: Report of a case. Pediatrics 16:857.

14. KURREIN, F. 1954. Cerebral mucormycosis. J. Clin. Path. 7:141.

15. LA TOUCHE, C. J., T. W. Sutherland and J. Telling. 1964. Histopathological and mycological features of a case of rhinocerebral mucormycosis (phycomycosis) in Britain. Sabouraudia, 3:148.

16. LIE-KIAN-JOE, N. T. E., A. Pahan and H. Van Der Muelen. 1956. *Basidiobolus ranarum* as a cause of subcutaneous mycosis in Indonesia. Arch. Dermat. 74:378.

17. MEAME, P., and D. Rayner. 1960. Mucormycosis. A report on twenty-two cases. Arch. Pathol. 70:261.

18. MOORE, M., W. A. D. Anderson and H. H. Everett. 1949. Mucormycosis of the large bowel. Am. J. Path. 25:559.

19. SAUER, R. M. 1966. Cutaneous mucormycosis (phycomycosis) in a squirrel *(Sciurus carolinensis)*. Am. J. Vet. Res. 27:380.

20. SCHOFIELD, R. A. and R. D. Baker. 1956. Experimental mucormycosis *(Rhizopus* infection) in mice. Arch. Path. 61:407.

21. SHIRLEY, A. G. H. 1965. Two cases of phycomycotic ulceration in sheep. Vet. Rec. 77:675.

22. SRINIVASAN, M. C. and M. J. Thirumalachar. 1965. *Basidiobolus* species pathogenic for man. Sabouraudia, 4:32.

23. VIGNALE, R., J. E. Mackinnon, E. C. Vilaboa and F. Burgoa. 1964. Chronic, destructive, mucocutaneous phycomycosis in man. Sabouraudia, 3:143.

24. WADSWORTH, J. A. C. 1951. Ocular mucormycosis: report of a case. Am. J. Ophth. 34:405.

PENICILLIOSIS

Definition:

In rare cases, penicilliosis has included pulmonary involvement, onychomycosis, otomycosis, and mycetomas, and has been considered to be due to the presence of various species of *Penicillium*. *Penicillium* strains along with other molds have been reported as excitants in some allergic bronchial asthma cases. A variety of *Penicillium* species may be agents of infection of the cornea. The closely related genus *Scopulariopsis* at times is the cause of onychomycosis and peronychia. Another closely related genus, *Paecilomyces,* has been reported as a cause of endocarditis.

Etiological Agents:

Various species of *Penicillium, Scopulariopsis brevicaulis* or *Paecilomyces*. For the diseases onychomycosis, otomycosis, and maduromycosis involving *Penicillium* refer to the respective disease for additional details on procedures.

Occurrence:

1. **Man:** *Penicillium* sp. have been reported in pulmonary infections from urine, bladder, and kidney in the United States; in otomycosis in many areas. *Scopulariopsis* sp. has been reported as a cause of nail infections and as the cause of an inguinal ulcer in the United States, and *Paecilomyces* sp. as a cause of endocarditis.

2. **Animals:** Genital mucosa and vaginal infections in bulls and cows have been reported in Germany, and *Penicillium marneffei* Segretain, 1959 has been reported as an unusual mycosis in bamboo rats, resembling *Histoplasma capsulatum* in the polymorphonuclear leukocytes, reticulocytes, and giant cells of the animals.

Laboratory Procedures

1. **Sources of Infected Material:** Infected nail or skin should be removed and placed in a sterile container. Other specimens such as sputum, urine, or biopsies should be put in sterile containers for examination in the laboratory.

2. **Examination of Infected Material:**

   a. Place nail or skin material on a slide with potassium hydroxide (see procedure for dermatophytes). Sputum or urine should be placed directly on a slide and a cover glass added.

   b. Microscopically, small, round conidia and fragments of septate hyphae should be found for *Penicillium* infections (this is similar to those seen for *Aspergillus).* Debris below the nail in an onychomycosis case should show numerous hyphae and round conidia if *Scopulariopsis* is the cause of the infections. *Scopulariopsis* may occur as an opportunistic pathogen.

3. **Cultures:**

   a. *Penicillium* sp. should be cultured on Czapek agar and other appropriate media for study of colony characteristics and identification. See section on contaminants for genus characteristics and *A Manual of the Penicillia* by Raper and Thom for species identification.

   b. *Scopulariopsis* sp. can be cultured on Sabouraud's glucose agar at room temperature. The fast-growing fungus produces a tan to brown powdery colony. See section on contaminants for characteristics of the genus. *Scopulariopsis brevicaulis* (Saccardo) Brainier, 1907, is the species usually isolated.

   c. *Paecilomyces* sp. can be cultured on Sabouraud glucose agar. See contaminant section for characteristics of genus.

NOTE: It is important to demonstrate the fungus in tissue sections if possible as well as in culture as repeated isolation of the organism from sputum or other sources of material from patients will not necessarily indicate the organism as the causative agent.

4. **Animal Inoculation:** No specific value.

Questions:

1. Why is it difficult to establish the etiological relationship of these organisms as causative agents of a disease?

2. List references that may be used in the identification of *Penicillium* sp., *Scopulariopsis* sp. and *Paecilomyces* sp.

Selected References

1. AIMÉ, P., P. Creuzé and H. Kresser. 1933. Mycose Pulmonaire. A *Penicillium crustaceum;* avec signes clinique d'abcès du Paumon. Presse Méd. 41:761.
2. GILLIAM, J. S. and S. A. Vest. 1951. *Penicillium* infection of the urinary tract. Jour. Urol. 65:484.
3. GRÉGOIRE, P. E., R. Linz and O. Van Damme. 1953. Apparitions successives d'un *Penicillium* et d'un *Aspergillus* dans un liquide pleural. Acta Clin. Belg. 8:483.
4. HUANG, S. N. and L. S. Harris. 1963. Acute disseminated penicilliosis. Report of a case and review of pertinent literature. Am. J. Clin. Path. 39:167.
5. JANKE, D. 1953. Scoplariopsisarten als menschenpathogene Dermatophyten. Z. Haut. u. Geschlkrankh. 14:35.
6. MARKLEY, A. J., O. S. Philpott and F. D. Weidman. 1936. Deep scopulariopsis of ulcerating granuloma type confirmed by culture and animal inoculation. Arch. Dermat. and Syph. 33:627.
7. MARTIN-SCOTT, I. 1954. Onychomycosis caused by *Scopulariopsis brevicaulis.* Trans. Brit. Mycol. Soc. 37:38.
8. NENCIONI, M. 1925. Onychomycosis caused by *Penicillium brevicaule.* Demart. Ztscher. 45:116.
9. NUSSBAUM, A. and T. Benedek. 1927. Penicilliosis in piano-factory worker. Beitr. z. Klin. Tuberk. 67:756.
10. PERRY, J. E. 1964. Opportunistic fungal infections of the urinary tract. Texas J. Med. 60:146.
11. RAPER, K. B. and C. Thom. 1949. A Manual of the Penicillia. Williams and Wilkins Co., Baltimore.
12. SEGRETAIN, G. 1959. *Penicillium marneffei* n. sp. agent d'une mycose du systeme reticuloendothelial. Mycopathologia 11:327.
13. SEGRETAIN, G. 1964. Formes parasitaires des histoplasmes et de *Penicillium marneffei.* Ann. Soc. Belge Méd. Trop. 44:331.
14. UYS, C. G., P. A. Don, V. Schrire and C. N. Barnard. 1963. Endocarditis following surgery due to the fungus *Paecilomyces.* South Afr. Med. J. 37:1276.

CLADOSPORIOSIS

Definition:

Cladosporiosis is caused by species of *Cladosporium*. Infections occur in most cases as brain abscesses, and occasionally as pulmonary lesions.

Etiological Agents:

The fungus usually causing most of the brain abscesses is *Cladosporium bantianum* (Sacc.) Borelli, 1960 (Synonymy: *Cladosporium trichoides* Emmons in Binford et al, 1952). Borelli (1960) considered *C. trichoides* to be the same as *C. bantianum,* although the spores of the latter are larger and borne in unbranched chains (Emmons, et al., 1963; Emmons, 1966). *Phialophora dermatitidis* and *Fonsecaea pedrosoi* have been reported as causative agents in several brain abscess cases.

Occurrence:

1. **Man:** Cases have been reported in North America, South America, Europe, India, Japan, and Africa.
2. **Animals:** No known cases.

Laboratory Procedures

1. **Source of Infected Material:** Biopsy of brain specimens or removal of material from brain abscesses, lung, or cutaneous skin ulcers should be kept in sterile containers for laboratory study.

2. **Examination of Infected Material:**

   a. Smears should be made of material from brain abscesses or dermal ulcers. The addition of KOH or lactophenol cotton blue should be satisfactory unless sufficient liquid is already present.

   b. Microscopically, hyphae are branched, septate, and brownish-yellow in color in tissue or pus. Individual spherical cells or moniliform chains may appear.

3. **Cultures:** The organism grows readily on Sabouraud glucose agar with or without antibiotics at 24° or 37° C (maximum up to 42° to 43° C). The colony develops as a spreading growth (about 4 cm in two weeks), with a velvety olive-gray to brown surface. Older colonies develop radial folds.

   Microscopically, septate, brown conidiophores develop (typical for *Cladosporium),* forming branched chains of conidia with the youngest cells forming by budding. Conidia are about 2-2.5 by 4-7 μ in size, separated in the chain by disjunctors.

4. **Biochemical Activities:** Strains of *C. bantianum* do not: liquefy gelatin or Loffler's coagulated serum, hydrolyze starch, coagulate milk, or utilize tributyrine and cellulose. The saprophytic species are positive for all these tests except tributyrine and cellulose.

5. **Animal Inoculation:** In mice, intravenous inoculations of 300,000 spores can be made to develop cerebral lesions. This may be useful for species identification. Mice should be autopsied after clinical signs of cerebral infection appear. Make slides for microscopic examination and culture parts of the brain.

Selected References

1. AL-DOORY, Y. and M. A. Gordon. 1963. Application of fluorescent-antibody procedures to the study of pathogenic dematiaceous fungi. I. Differentiation of *Cladosporium carrionii* and *Cladosporium bantianum.* J. Bact. 86:332.

2. BAGCHI, A., B. K. Aikat and D. Barua. 1962. Granulomatous lesion of the brain produced by *Cladosporium trichoides.* J. Indian Med. Assoc. 38:602.

3. BINFORD, C. H., R. K. Thompson, M. E. Gorham and C. W. Emmons. 1952. Mycotic brain abscess due to *Cladosporium trichoides,* a new species. Am. J. Clin. Path. 22:535.

4. BORELLI, D. 1960. *Torula bantiana,* agente di un granuloma cerebrale. Riv. Anat. Patrol Oncol. 17:617.

5. DESAI, S. C., M. L. Bhatikar and R. S. Mehta. 1966. Cerebral chromblastomycosis due to *Cladosporium trichoides (Bantianum).* Part II. Neurology India 14:8.

6. DUQUE, O. 1961. Meningo-encephalitis and brain abscess caused by *Cladosporium* and *Fonsecaea.* Am. J. Clin. Path. 36:505.

7. EMMONS, C. W. 1966. Pathogenic dematiaceous fungi. Jap. J. Med. Mycol. 7:233.

8. KING, A. B. and T. S. Collette. 1952. Brain abscess due to *Cladosporium trichoides.* Bull. Johns Hopkins Hosp. 91:298.

9. RILEY, O., Jr. and S. H. Mann. 1960. Brain abscess caused by *Cladosporium trichoides.* Am. J. Clin. Path. 33:525.

10. SHIMAZONO, Y., I. Kiminori, H. Torii, R. Otsuka and T. Fukushiro. 1963. Brain abscess due to *Hormodendrum dermatidis* (Kano) Conant 1953. Report of a case and review of the literature. Folia Psychiat. Neurol. Jap. 17:80.

KERATOMYCOSIS

(Mycotic Infections of the Cornea)

Definition:

Fungus infection of the cornea is usually initiated by trauma. A white plaque develops after the spores germinate, and mycelial growth occurs in the area of the trauma. Ulceration develops in the cornea around the opacities. Another condition known as histoplasma uveitis may develop in the eye, and other fungal invasions of the eye may occur.

Etiological Agents:

Many different fungi may be the etiological agents of keratomycosis. These may include some yeastlike species of *Candida* to many other fungi that are often soil saprophytes. Examples of some genera isolated from corneal scrapings are: *Aspergillus* sp., *Cephalosporium* sp., *Cladosporium* sp., *Curvularia* sp., *Fusarium* sp., *Monosporium* sp., *Penicillium* sp., *Scopulariopsis* sp., etc. The organism *Histoplasma capsulatum* has not been demonstrated for histoplasma uveitis at the present time.

Occurrence:

1. **Man:** Worldwide in distribution. The incidence of mycotic infections of the cornea has increased following the use of antibiotics or topical cortisones.

2. **Animals:** Intracorneal necrosis in the rabbit eye has been established under laboratory conditions.

Laboratory Procedures

1. **Source of Infected Material:** Scrapings should be taken deep in the ulceration around the opacities for laboratory examination and culture.

2. **Examination of Infected Material:**

   a. Corneal scrapings of the filamentous fungi in 10% KOH or lactophenol should appear as septate, branching, hyphal fragments. For *Candida* sp., pseudohyphae or budding cells will be seen.

3. **Cultures:** Sabouraud glucose agar with chloramphenicol is suitable for most of the organisms likely to be isolated. The infected material should be placed on the medium and kept at 24° C. For a description of the etiological agents listed above, see references on other pages in this manual or other books.

4. **Histopathology:** Sections of the eye should be stained with PAS, Gridley, or the Gomori methamine silver stain. In the PAS and Gridley stained sections, the fungal structures will appear red, while in the Gomori methenamine silver stain the structures will be black.

5. **Animal Inoculation:** Corneal infections have been established in rabbits by the use of cortisone and oxytetracycline or following trauma and inoculation of the organism.

Selected References

1. ANDERSON, B., Jr., S. S. Roberts, C. Gonzalez and E. W. Chick. 1959. Mycotic ulcerative keratitis. Arch. Ophthal. 62:169.

2. BERSON, E. L., G. S. Kobayashi and R. B. Oglesby. 1965. Treatment of experimental fungal keratitis. Archs. Ophthal. 74:403.

3. CHICK, E. W., and N. F. Conant. 1962. Mycotic ulcerative keratitis; a review of 148 cases from the literature (abstr). Invest. Ophthal. 1:419.

4. ERNEST, J. T. and J. W. Rippon. 1966. Keratitis due to *Allescheria boydii (Monosporium apiospermum)*. Amer. J. Ophthal. 62:1202.

5. FINE, B. S. 1962. Intraocular mycotic infections. Lab. Invest. 11:1161.

6. GINGRICH, W. D. 1962. Keratomycosis. J. Am. Med. Assoc. 179:649.

7. HAMMEKE, J. C. and P. P. Ellis. 1960. Mycotic flora of the conjunctiva. Amer. J. Ophthal. 49:1174. 1960.

8. LEY, A. P. and T. E. Sanders. 1956. Experimental fungus infections of the cornea; a preliminary report. Amer. J. Ophthal. 42:59.

9. MENDELBLATT, D. L. 1953. Moniliasis. A review and a report of the first case demonstrating the *Candida albicans* in the cornea. Am. J. Ophthal. 36:379.

10. MITSUI, Y. and J. Hanabusa. 1955. Corneal infections after cortisone therapy. Brit. J. Ophthal. 39:244.

11. NEMA, H. V., O. P. Ahuja and L. N. Mohapatra. 1966. Mycotic flora of the conjunctiva. Am. J. Ophthal. 62:968.

12. RHEINS, M. S., P. A. Pixley, T. Suie and R. H. Keates. 1966. Diagnosis of experimental fungal corneal ulcers by fluorescent antibody techniques. Am. J. Ophthal. 62:892.

13. SALFELDER, K. J. and M. Akbarian. 1965. Experimental ocular histoplasmosis in dogs. Am. J. Ophthal. 59:290.

14. SEGAL, P. 1968. Grzybicze choroby oka. (Fungal eye diseases). 155 pp. 64 fig. Warszawa. Panstwowy Zaklad Wydawnictw Lekarskich.

15. SUIE, T. and W. H. Havener. 1963. Mycology of the eye: a review. Amer. J. Ophthal. 56:63.

16. ZIMMERMAN, L. E. 1962. Mycotic keratitis. Lab. Invest. 11:1151.

SOURCES FOR MEDIA, CULTURES, EQUIPMENT AND VISUAL AIDS

The following list contains some of the sources where materials may be procured for courses and laboratory work in medical mycology:

1. Baltimore Biological Laboratory (BBL), Division of BioQuest, P.O. Box 175, Cockeysville, Md. 21030.

2. Bioquest, P.O. Box 243, Cockeysville, Md. 21030.

3. Calbiochem, 3625 Medford St., Los Angeles, Calif. 90063.

4. Central Scientific Co., 2600 S. Kostner Ave., Chicago, Ill. 60623.

5. Clay-Adams, 299 Webro Rd., Parsippany, N. J. 07054.

6. Colab Laboratories, Inc., 3 Science Road, Glenwood, Ill. 60425.

7. Difco Laboratories, Inc., 920 Henry St., Detroit, Mich. 48201.

8. Eberbach Corp., 505 S. Maple Rd., Ann Arbor, Mich. 48106.

9. Fisher Scientific Co., 711 Forbes Ave., Pittsburg, Pa. 15219.

10. Greiner Scientific Corporation, 22 N. Moore St., New York, N. Y. 10013.

11. Hyland Division of Travenol Laboratories, Inc., 3300 Hyland Ave., Costa Mesa, Calif. 92626.

12. Lederle Laboratories, Clinical Laboratory Aids Department, Pearl River, N. Y. 10965.

13. Mann Research Laboratories, Division of Becton, Dickinson and Co., Mountain View Ave., Orangeburg, N. Y. 10962.

14. Matheson Coleman and Bell, P.O. Box 85, East Rutherford, N. J. 07073.

15. Matheson Scientific, 1850 Greenleaf Ave., Elk Grove Village, Ill. 60007.

16. Nutritional Biochemicals Corporation, 26201 Miles Rd., Cleveland, Ohio 44128.

17. Pfizer Diagnostics Division, Chas. Pfizer and Co., Inc., 300 W. 43rd St., New York, N. Y. 10036.

18. Sargent-Welch Co., 4647 W. Foster Ave., Chicago, Ill. 60630.

19. Scientific Products, 1210 Leon Place, Evanston, Ill. 60201.

20. Sigma Chemical Co., 3500 DeKalb St., St. Louis, Mo. 63118.

21. Arthur H. Thomas Co., P.O. Box 779, Vine St. at Third, Philadelphia, Pa. 19105.

Cultures

Some of the pathogenic fungi may be secured from the following concerns:

1. American Type Culture Collection, 12301 Parklawn Drive, Rockville, Maryland 20852.

2. Carolina Biological Supply Co., Burlington, North Carolina 27216.

3. Centraalbureau Voor Schimelcultures, Oosterstraat 1, Baarn (Netherlands).

4. General Biological Supply House (Turtox), 8200 South Hoyne Avenue, Chicago, Ill. 60620.

5. Hospital laboratories and universities where cultures of the various pathogenic fungi are maintained.

6. Department of Health, Education and Welfare, Public Realth Service, National Communicable Disease Center, Atlanta, Georgia 30333.

Visual Aids

1. <u>Movies</u>.
   a. The following films are available on a short term rental basis from the American Society for Microbiology, 1913 I St., N.W., Washington, D.C. 20006.

      (1) The diagnosis and management of Cutaneous Blastomycosis (Gilchrist's disease).

      (2) The Treatment of Moniliasis with Nystatin.

      (3) Mississippi Valley Disease — Histoplasmosis.

   b. The Department of Medical Communications, University of Kansas Medical Center, Rainbow Boulevard at 39th St., Kansas City, Kansas 66103, has the following films:

      (1) An Epidemic of Histoplasmosis

      (2) North American Blastomycosis

   c. Association Films, Inc., 512 Burlington Ave., La Grange, Illinois 60525 has the following film:

      (a) Treatment of Moniliasis with Nystatin.

   d. The Association Films, Inc., 561 Hillgrove Avenue, LaGrange, Ill. 60525, has the following film available:

      (1) Griseofulvin, Treatment of Superficial Fungus Infection.

      (2) Fungus Infections of the Foot.

   e. National Medical Audiovisual Center (Annex), Chamblee, Georgia 30005 has the following film for loan:

      (1) Coccidioidomycosis, Its Epidemiologic and Clinical Aspects, (M-175).

      (2) Histoplasmosis, Mason City, Iowa (M-1228).

      (3) Isolation of *Blastomyces Dermatitidis* (M-991).

      (4) Isolation of *Coccidioides Immitis* (M-990).

2. <u>Film Strips</u>. A catalog as well as film strips are available. The film strips requests should be sent to National Medical Audiovisual Center (Annex), Chamblee, Georgia 30005.

a. A Mycological Slide Culture Technique, (F-24).

b. Common Saprophytic Fungi, (F-446).

c. Laboratory Diagnosis of Ringworm in Animals. Part 1. *Microsporum* Infections, (F-221).

d. Laboratory Diagnosis of Ringworm in Animals. Part 2: *Trichophyton* Infections, (F-221a).

e. Laboratory Diagnosis of Tinea Capitis in Children: *Microsporum* Infections, (5-127).

f. Laboratory Diagnosis of *Trichophyton* Infections. Part 1: Ectothrix Infections of Beard and Scalp, (F-94a).

g. Laboratory Diagnosis of *Trichophyton* Infections. Part 2: Endothrix Infections of The Scalp, (F-94b).

h. *Blastomyces dermatitidis,* (F-116a).

i. *Coccidioides immitis,* (F-116b).

GLOSSARY

AEROBIC: requiring the presence of oxygen to grow.

ALEURIOSPORE: a lateral or terminal spore, well-attached to a conidiophore, detached by breaking of conidiophore wall.

ANAEROBIC: living in the absence of oxygen.

ANTHERIDIUM: male gametangium.

ARTHROSPORE: an asexual spore resulting from segmentation of a hypha.

ASCOGONIUM: a female gametangium.

ASCOSPORE: a spore formed as a result of sexual reproduction developed in a saclike cell known as an ascus.

ASCUS: a saclike structure containing usually 8 ascospores developed during sexual reproduction in the Ascomycetes.

ASEPTATE: lacking cross-walls.

ASEXUAL: reproduction in an organism without nuclear fusion.

BASIDIOSPORE: a spore borne on the outside of a basidium as a result of sexual reproduction in the Basidiomycetes.

BASIDIUM: a club-shaped structure bearing basidiospores.

BLASTOSPORE: a spore formed by budding from the hypha or somatic cell.

CHLAMYDOSPORE: a hyphal cell with a thick wall, becoming separated from the hypha and functioning as a spore.

CLAVATE: club-shaped structure.

CLEISTOTHECIUM: a closed ascocarp or fruiting body containing scattered asci.

COLUMELLA: a sterile structure usually in a sporangium or an extension of the sporangiophore.

CONIDIOPHORE: a specialized hypha bearing conidia.

CONIDIUM: an asexual spore produced at the tip or side of the conidiophore, or hypha.

DIMORPHIC: having two forms.

ECHINULATE: spiny.

ECTOTHRIX: a fungus which grows on the outside and inside of the hair shaft.

ENDOSPORE: an asexual spore formed within the cell.

ENDOTHRIX: a fungus which grows inside the hair shaft.

FAVIC CHANDELIERS: a group of irregular, broad, terminal hyphal branches with rounded ends, resembling antlerlike branches.

FAVIFORM: a convoluted or honeycomblike appearance in some colonies.

FISSION: division of cell into two cells by splitting.

FLOCCOSE: woolly appearance on the colony surface.

FRAGMENTATION: breaking or segmenting of the hypha each of which is capable of forming a new organism.

FLUORESCENCE: emitting light of a characteristic color from certain fungi when exposed to filtered ultraviolet light.

FUSEAU: a fusiform or spindle-shaped, multiseptate macroconidium.

FUSIFORM: a spindle-shaped structure tapering at the ends.

GLABROUS: smooth.

HYPHA: a branching tubular or threadlike structure of the fungi.

MACROCONIDIUM: a large, multi-celled conidium (fuseau).

MICROCONIDIUM: a small, usually one-celled conidium.

MICRON: a unit of measurement equal to one-thousandth part of a milimeter (0.001 mm.).
MURIFORM: a multi-celled, transverse and longitudinal septate conidium.
MYCELIUM: a mass of hyphae forming the vegetative portion of the thallus (body) of the fungus.
MYCOSIS: a disease produced by a fungus.

NODULAR BODY: one or more closely intertwined hyphae forming a rounded structure.

PECTINATE BODY: hyphal branch that is like a comb with parallel projections along one side.
PERITHECIUM: a closed ascocarp with an ostiole at the top, containing asci arranged in a layer
    inside.
PLEOMORPHISM: the occurrence of one or more forms in the life cycle of an organism, in many
    cases with reduced sporulation.
PYRIFORM: pear-shaped.

RACQUET HYPHA: enlarged, club-shaped hypha with the smaller end attached to the larger end
    of an adjacent club-shaped hypha.
RADIATE: to spread from a center.

SCUTULUM: cup-shaped crusts characteristic of favus, which usually is a fungus infection of the
    scalp.
SEPTATE: cross-walls in hypha.
SESSILE: attached directly by the base without a stalk.
SPIRAL HYPHA: coiled or corkscrewlike turns in a hypha.
SPORANGIOPHORE: a special hypha or stalk bearing a sporangium.
SPORANGIUM: a sac or cell containing one or more spores, usually produced asexually.
SPORE: a small reproductive unit or body, functioning like a seed, produced by the organism.
SPOROPHORE: any special structure bearing spores.
STERIGMA: a specialized hypha which supports a sporangium, a conidium, or basidiospore.

THALLUS: the vegetative or somatic portion of a fungus.
TINEA: ringworm or a skin disease caused by a fungus.

VERTICILLATE: structures arranged in whorls.
VESICLE: a blister or bladderlike structure.

ZYGOSPORE: a thick-walled spore formed by the fusion of two gametangia or specialized hyphae
    in the Phycomycetes.

INDEX